Exercises in Radiological Diagnosis

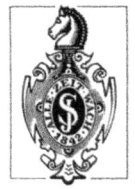

Pierre Bourjat

Radiology of the Hand

147 Radiological Exercises for Students and
Practitioners

With 284 Illustrations

Springer-Verlag Berlin Heidelberg GmbH

Professor PIERRE BOURJAT

Hospices Civils de Strasbourg
Centre Hospitalier Régional
1, Place de l'Hôpital
F-67091 Strasbourg

Translated from the French by

MARIE-THÉRÈSE WACKENHEIM

Library of Congress Cataloging in Publication Data. Bourjat, Pierre. Radiology of the hand. (Exercises in radiological diagnosis) Translation of: La main. Includes index. 1. Hand–Radiography–Problems, exercises, etc. 2. Hand–Diseases–Diagnosis–Problems, exercises, etc. I. Title. II. Series. [DNLM: 1. Hand–radiography–examination questions. WE 18 B774m] RC951.B6813   1987   617′.57507′57   86-22108

ISBN 978-3-540-16537-8   ISBN 978-3-662-02498-0 (eBook)
DOI 10.1007/978-3-662-02498-0

© Springer-Verlag Berlin Heidelberg 1987
Originally published by Springer-Verlag Berlin Heidelberg New York in 1987

2127/3130-543210

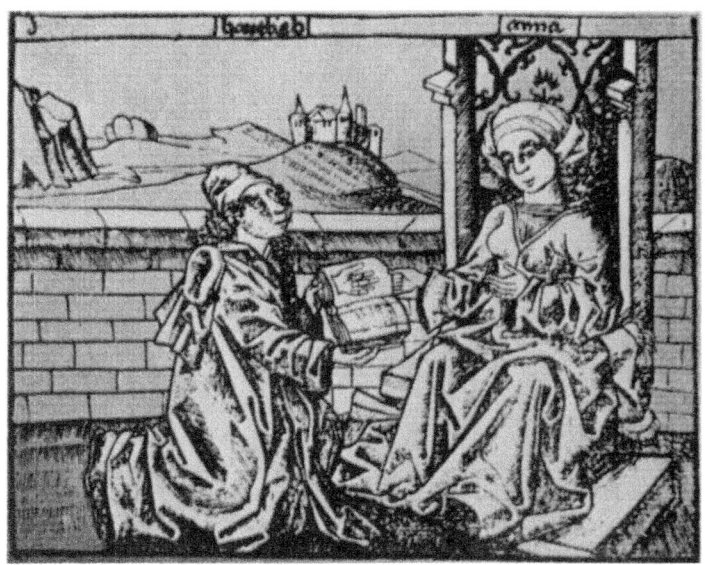

Johannes Hartlieb, physician in Vienna, gives with dedication
in 1448 his "Buch von der Hand" to duchess Anna of Bavaria.

Preface

I am proud that this study of the hand appears in the series Exercises in Radiological Diagnosis founded by A. WACKEN-HEIM.

From time eternal, man has tried to explain the numerous configurations and lines of the hand in order to reveal the true character of a person and to display his life. The importance of the symbolism of the hand is reflected in its role in the cultural life of the old world. Therefore, it is not astonishing that the first book about the hand, by Johannes Hartlieb, was devoted to Chiromancy, and that it was so successful that it went through four editions since the second half of the fifteenth century.

When Wilhelm Röntgen in 1895 asked his wife to lay her hand on a photographic plate covered with black paper and exposed it to the radiation he had just discovered, it marked the beginning of radiology. Today the study of the hand concerns only 2%–4% of the activity of radiology. It nevertheless reveals an amazing quantity and variety of pathology. That is the reason for this work.

The authors wishes to thank his friends Y. DIRHEIMER, rheumatologist, J. C. DOSCH, traumatologist, and G. FOUCHER, surgeon, who provided some of the material for the illustrations.

P. BOURJAT

Contents

Part One

Iconography

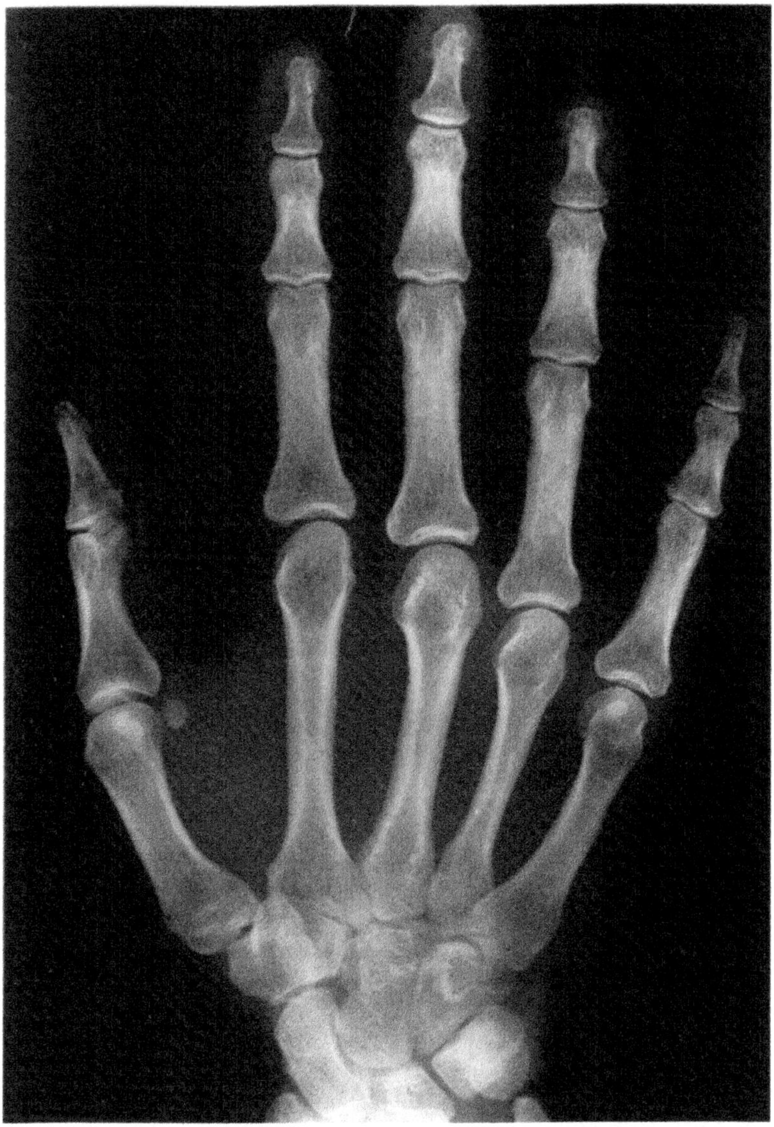

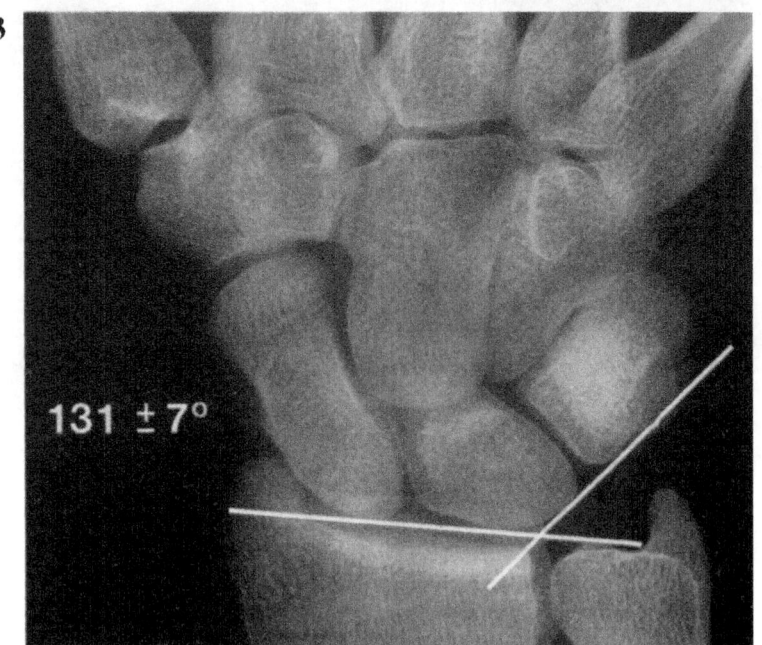

2

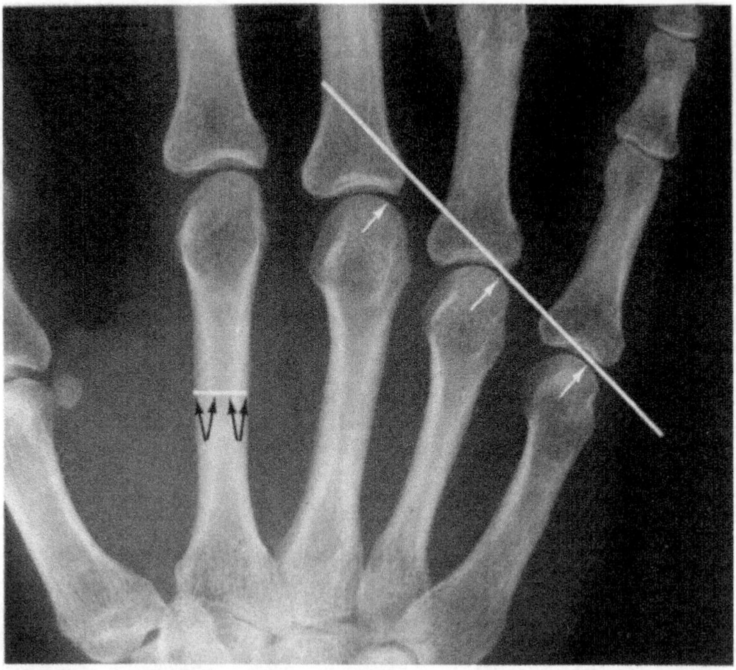

3

131 ± 7°

4

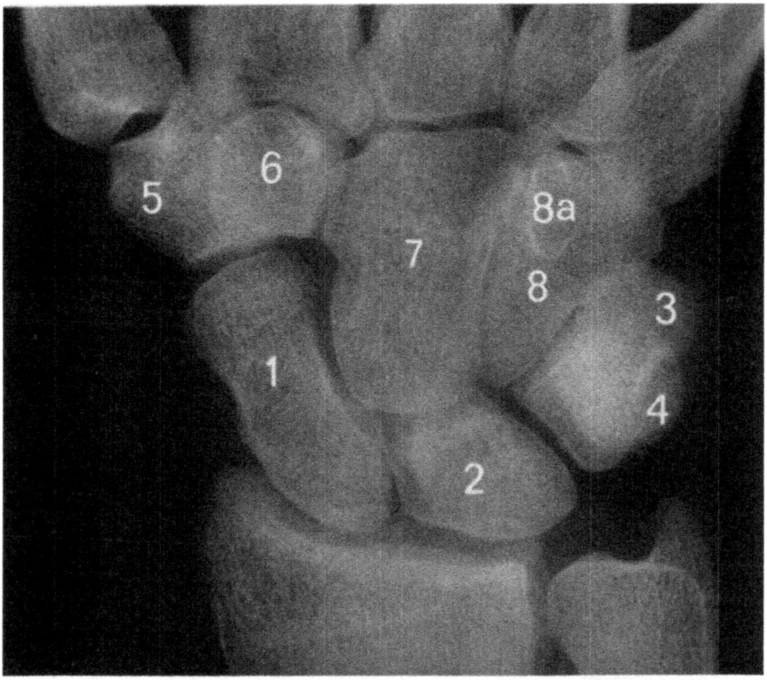

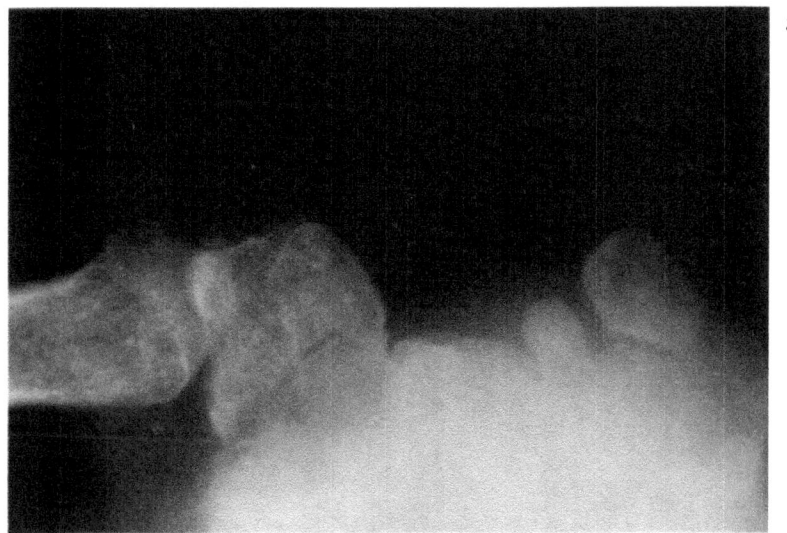

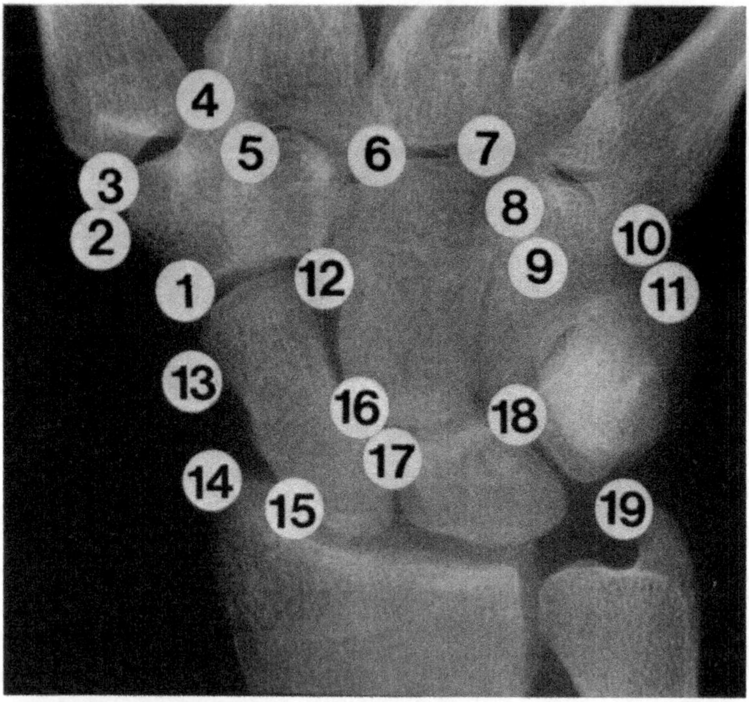

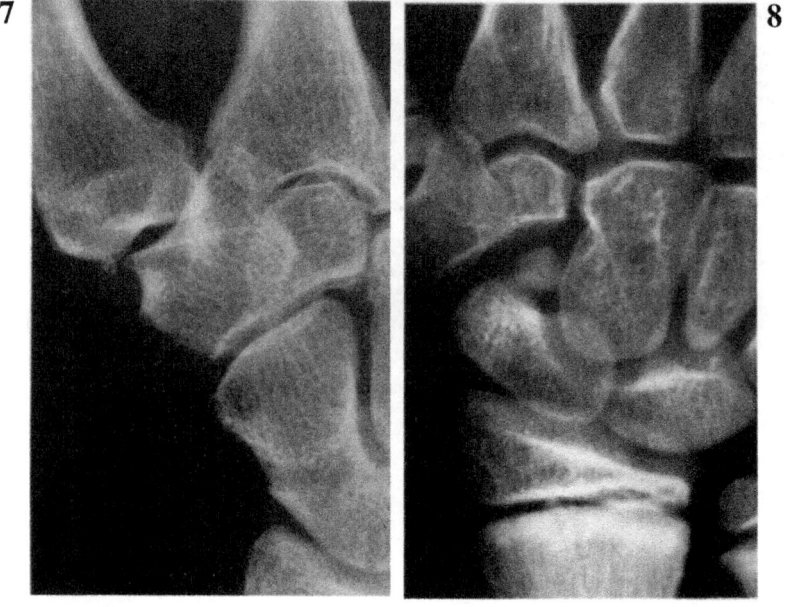

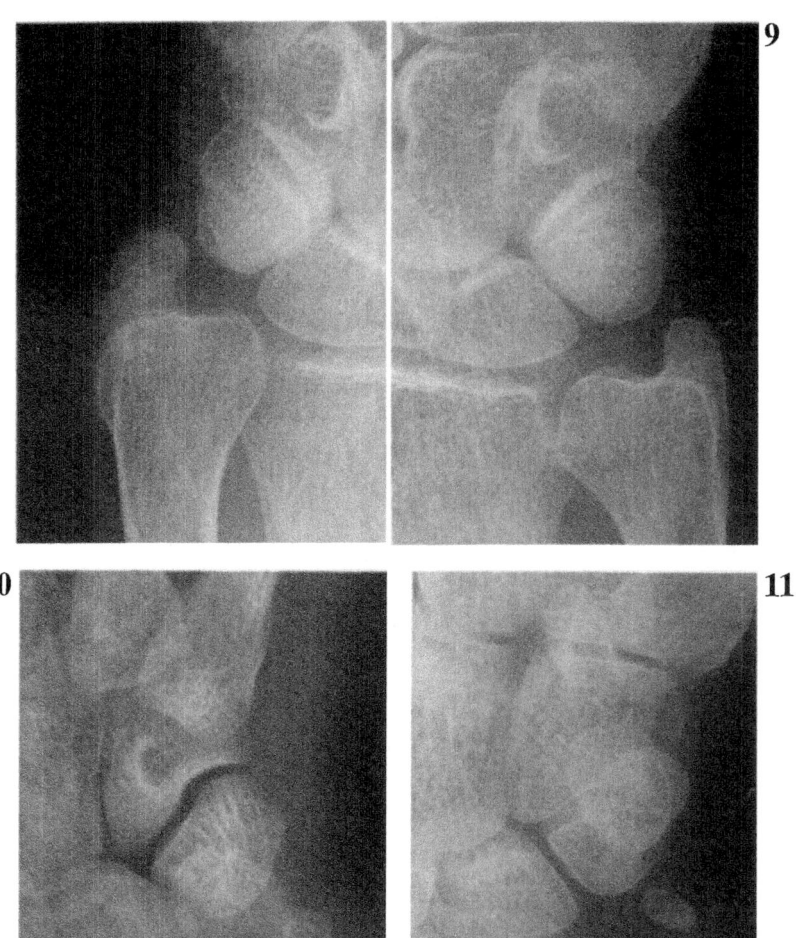

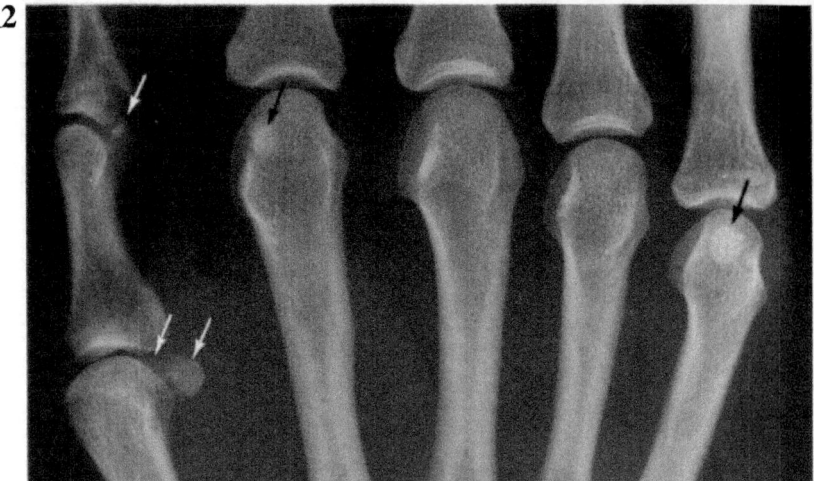

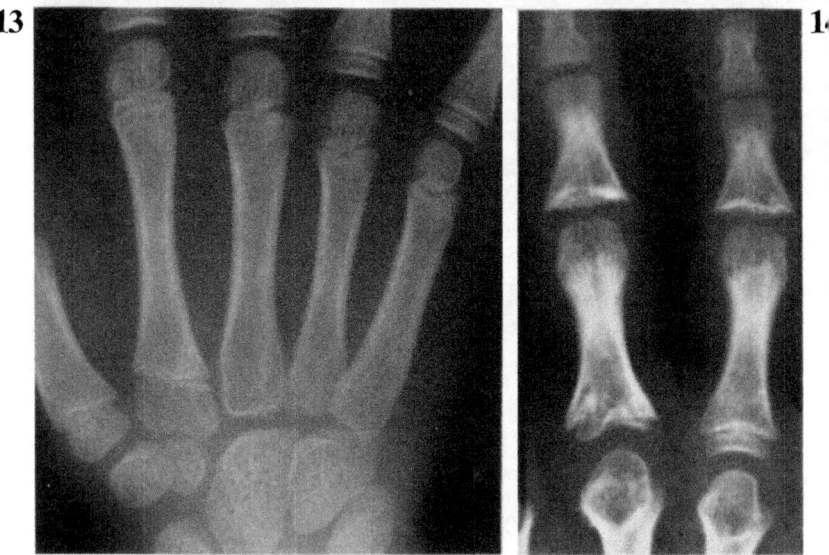

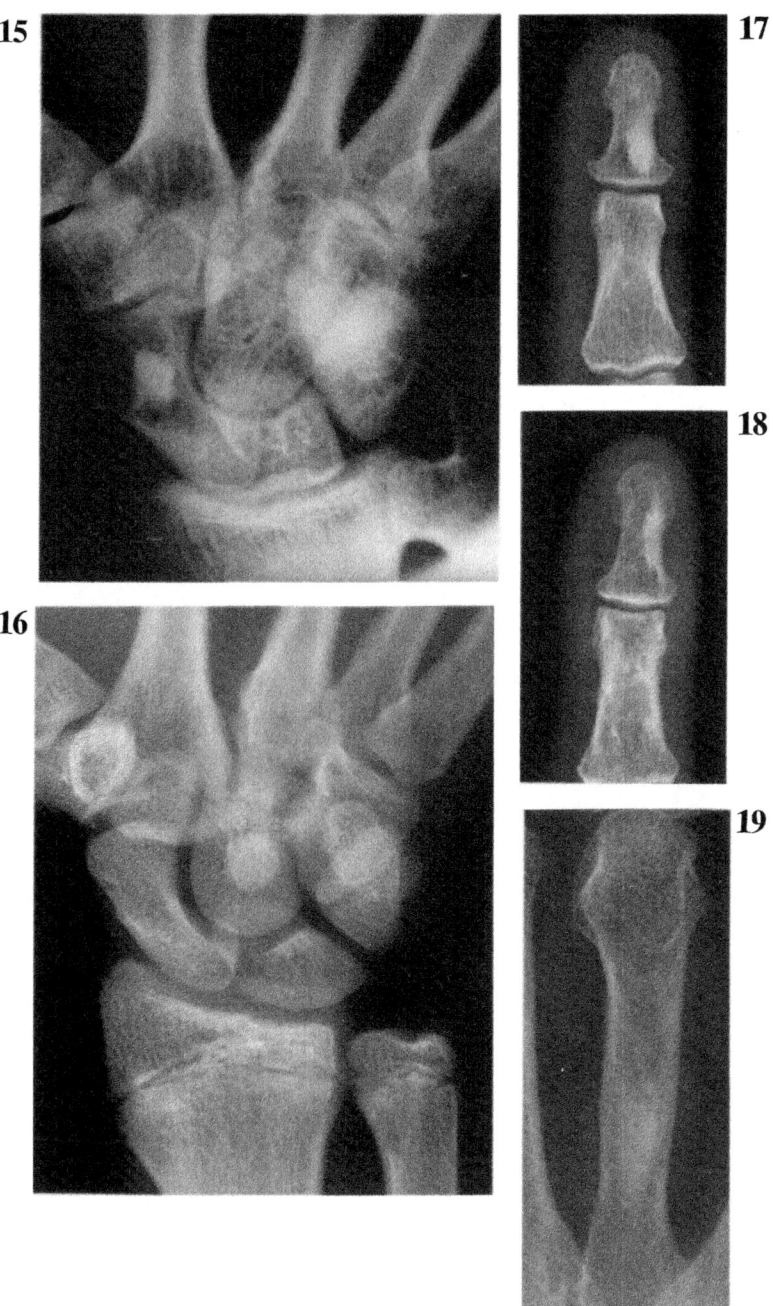

20

21

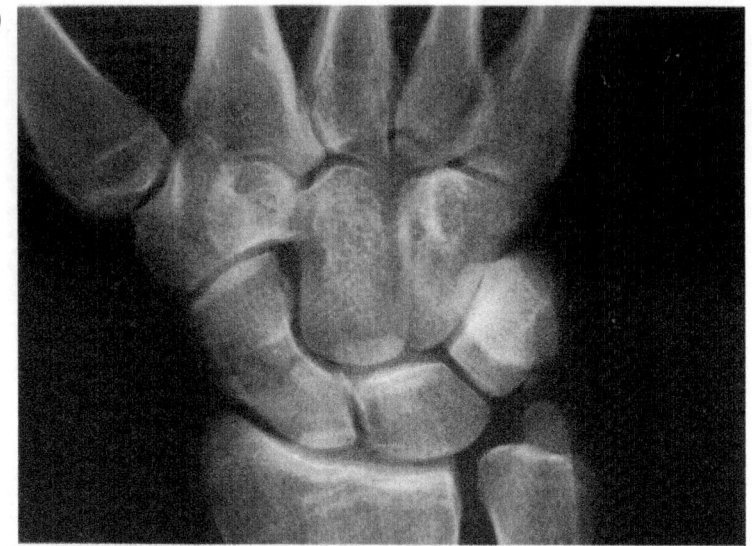

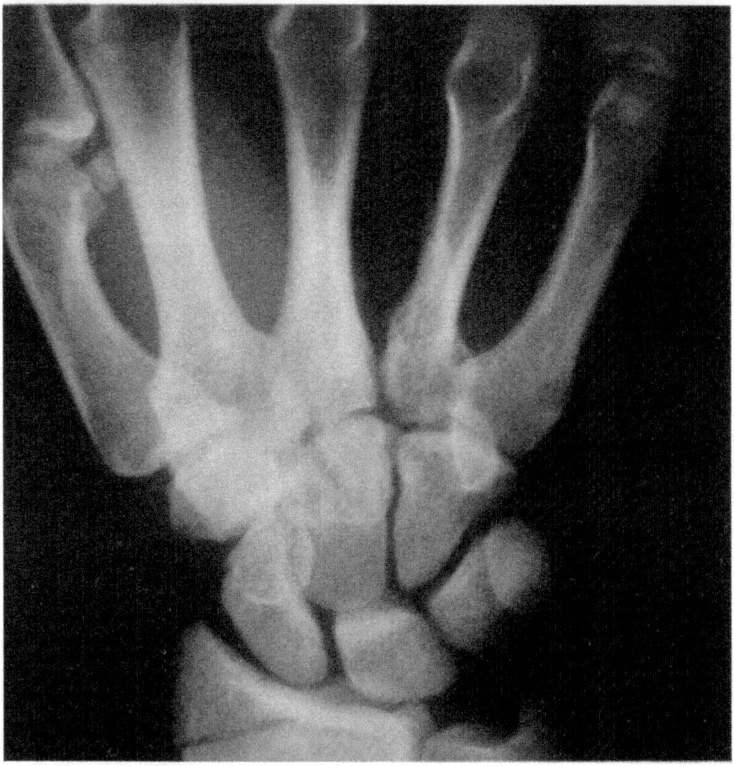

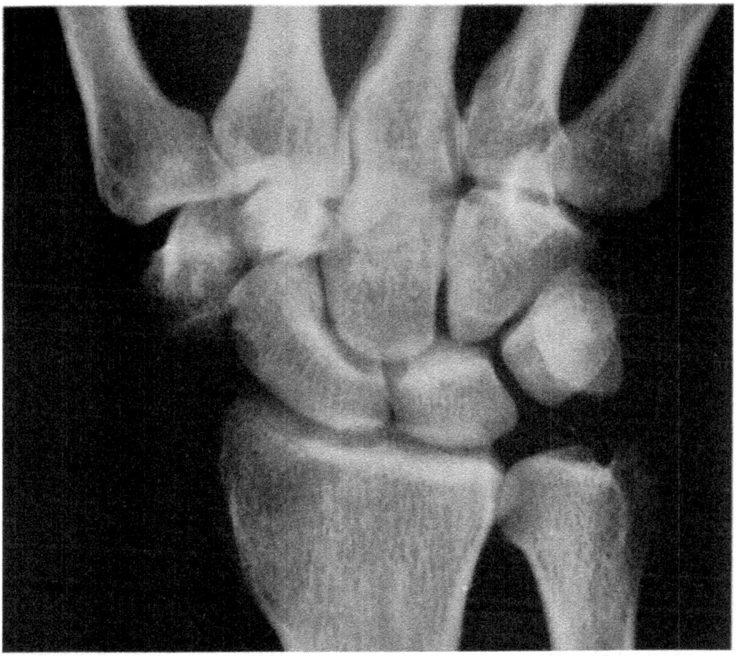

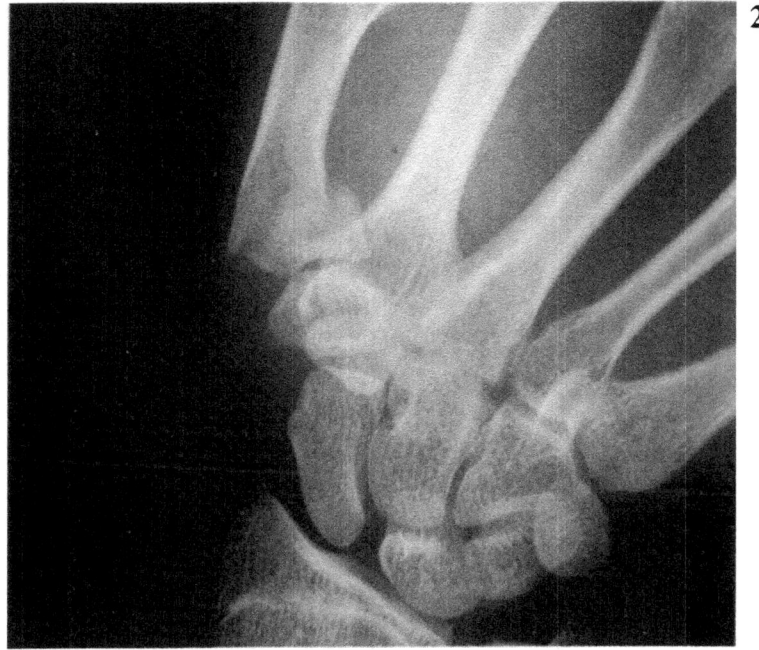

22

23

24

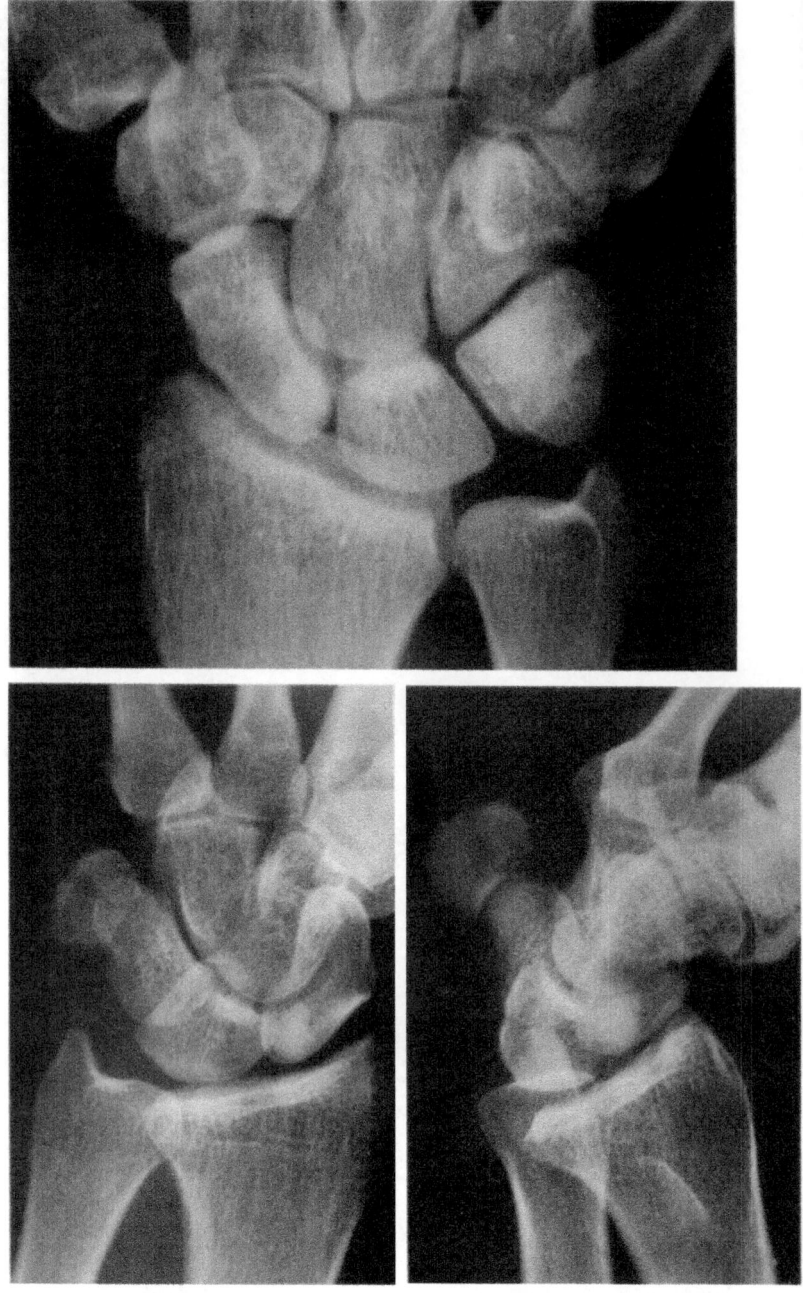

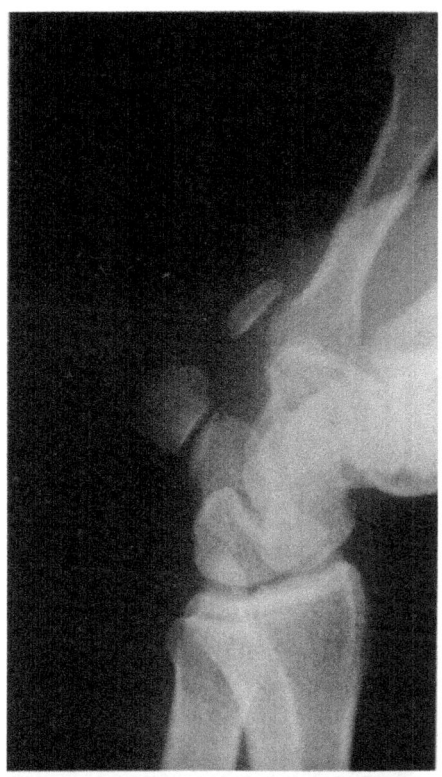

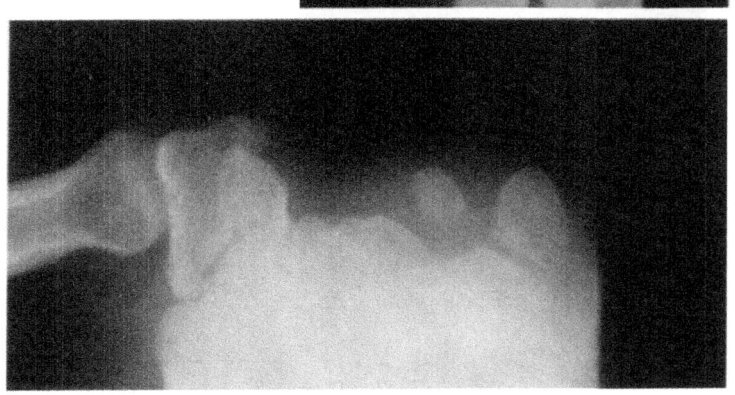

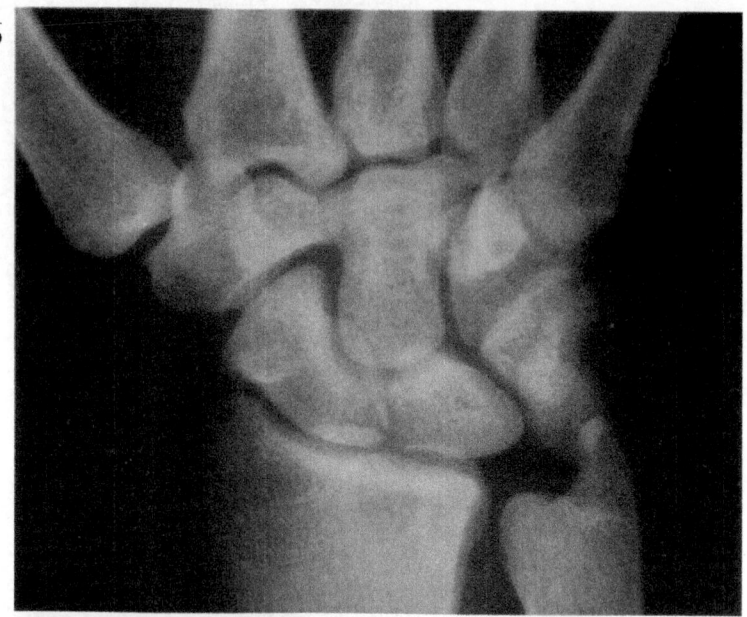

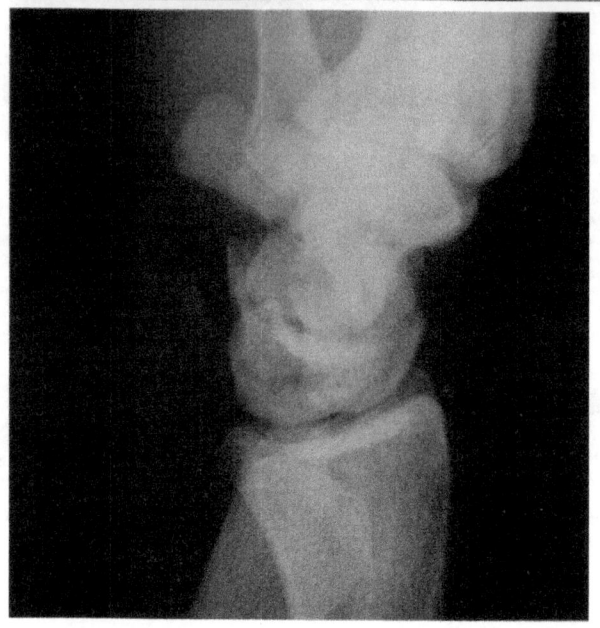

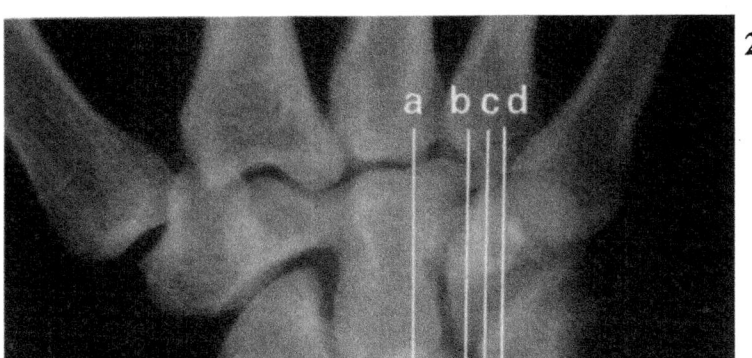

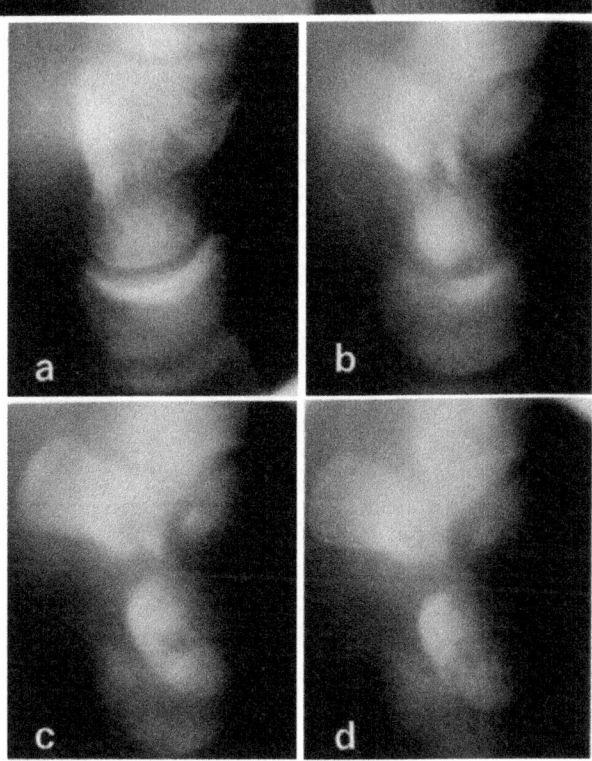

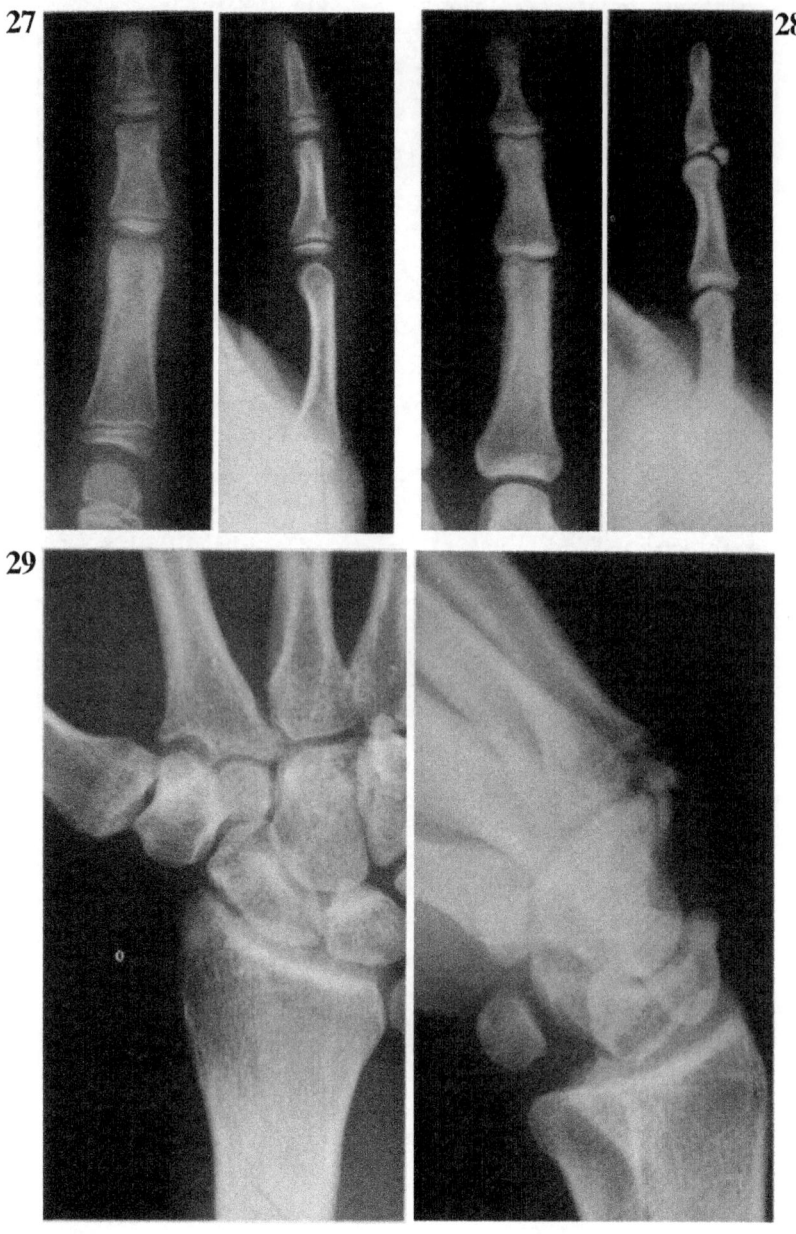

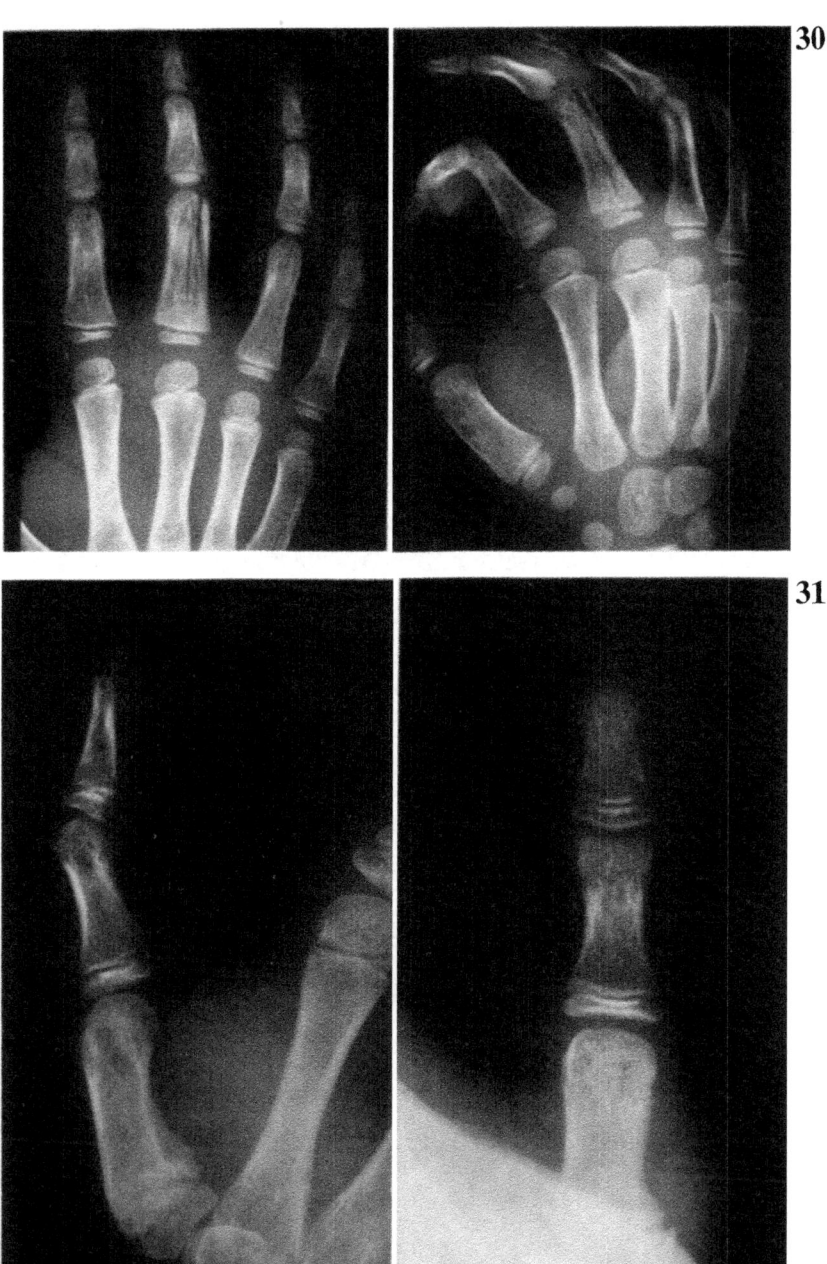

32

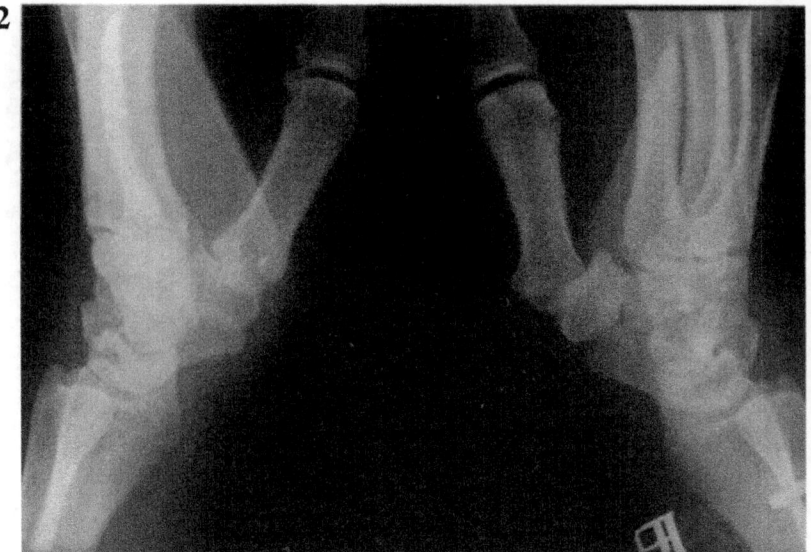

33

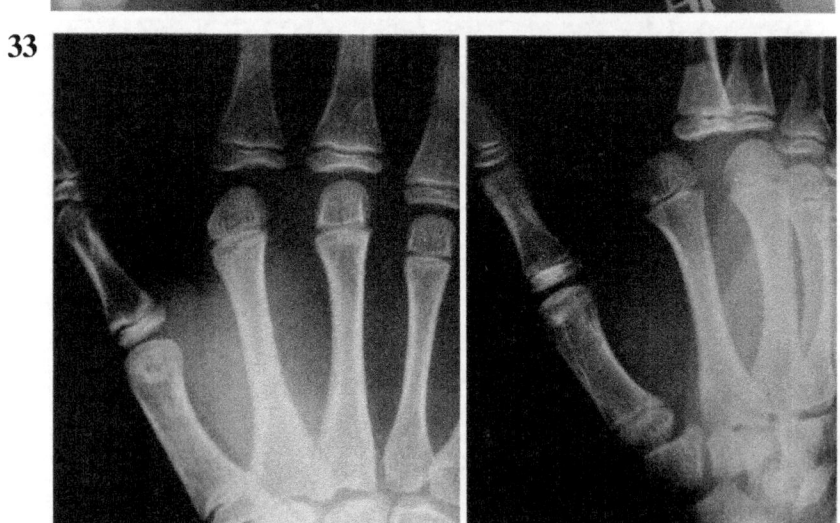

18

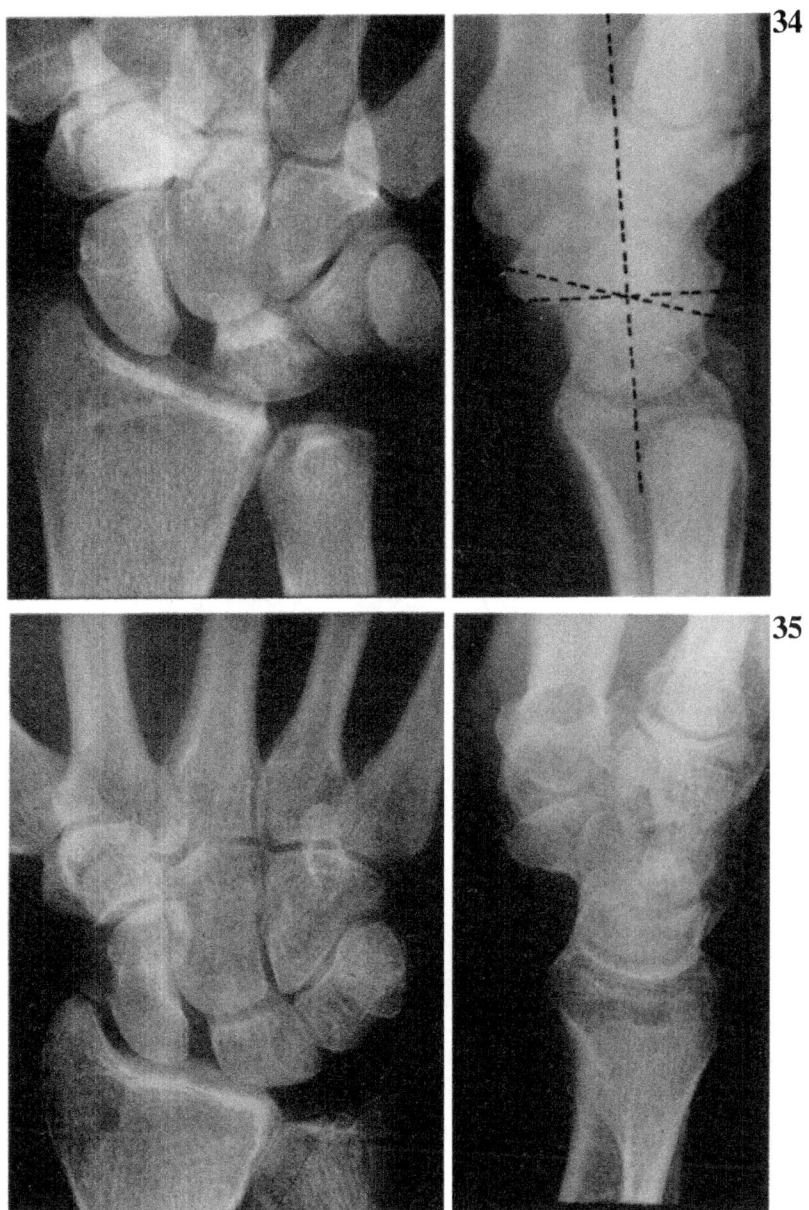

34

35

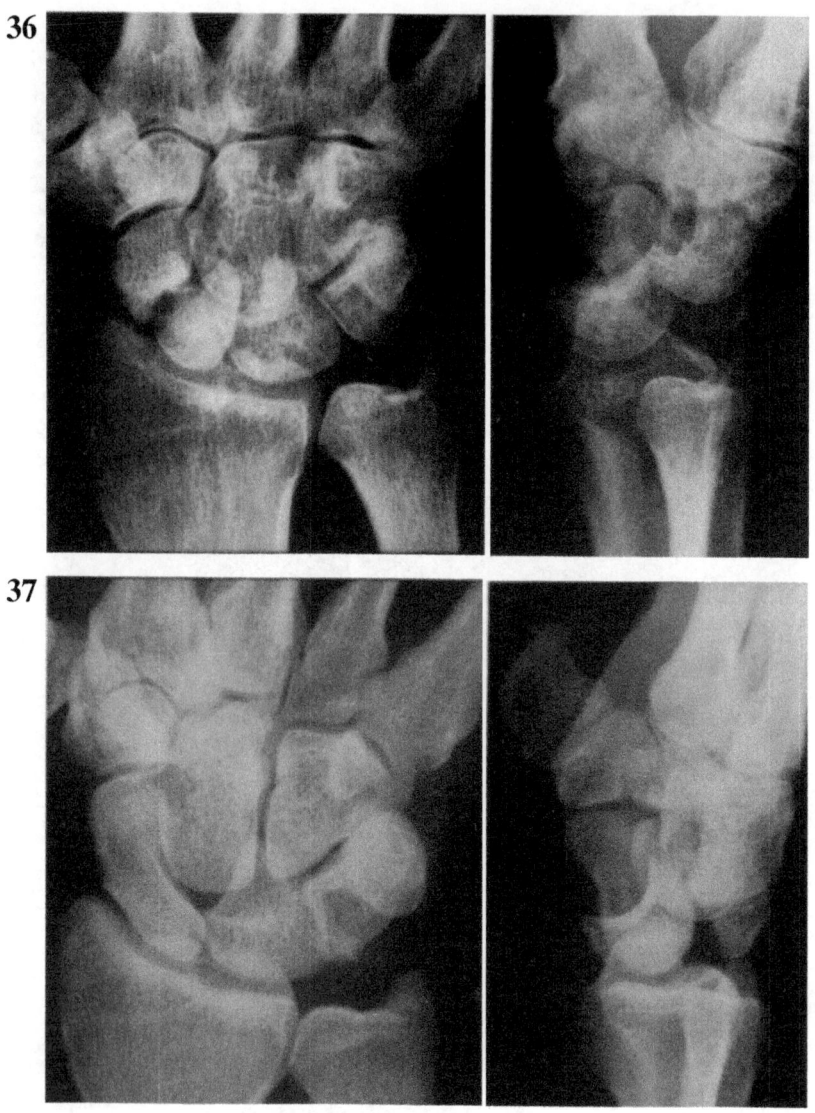

36

37

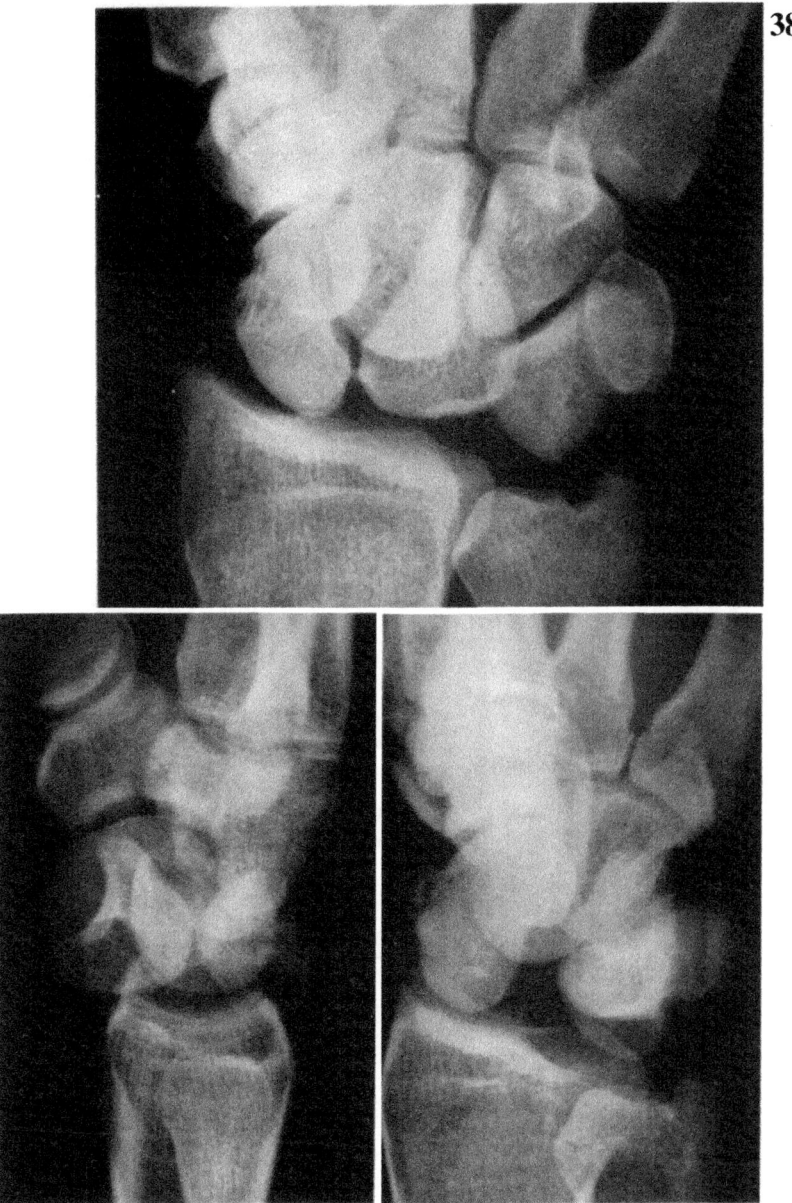

39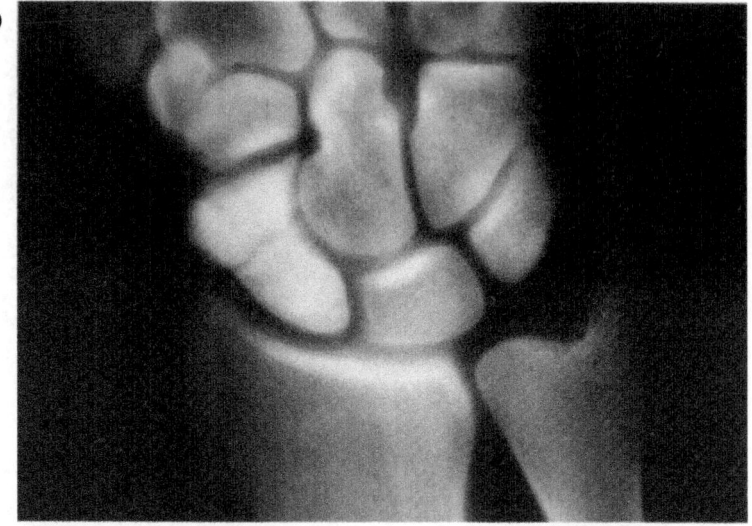

40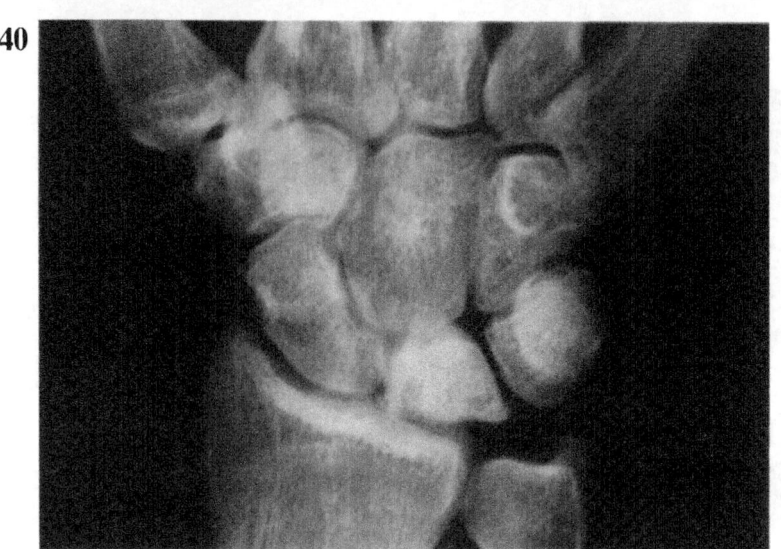

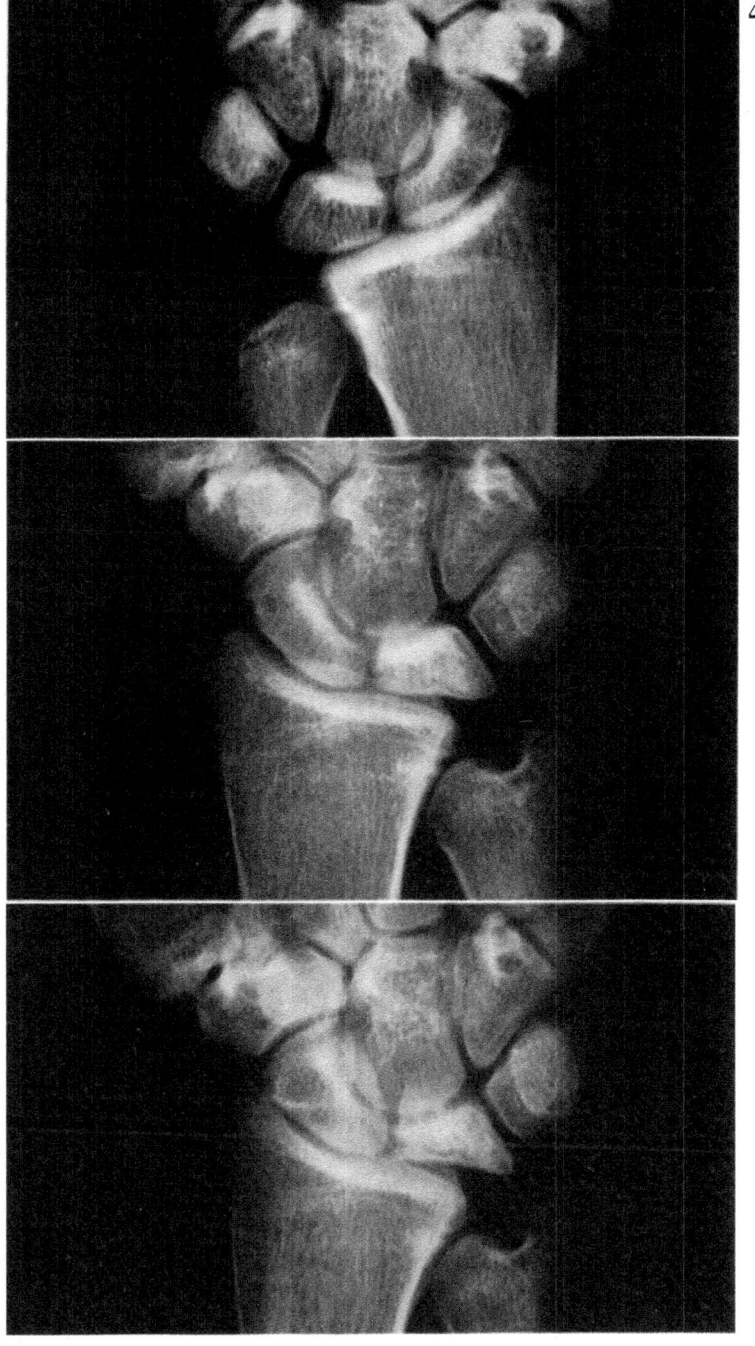

42

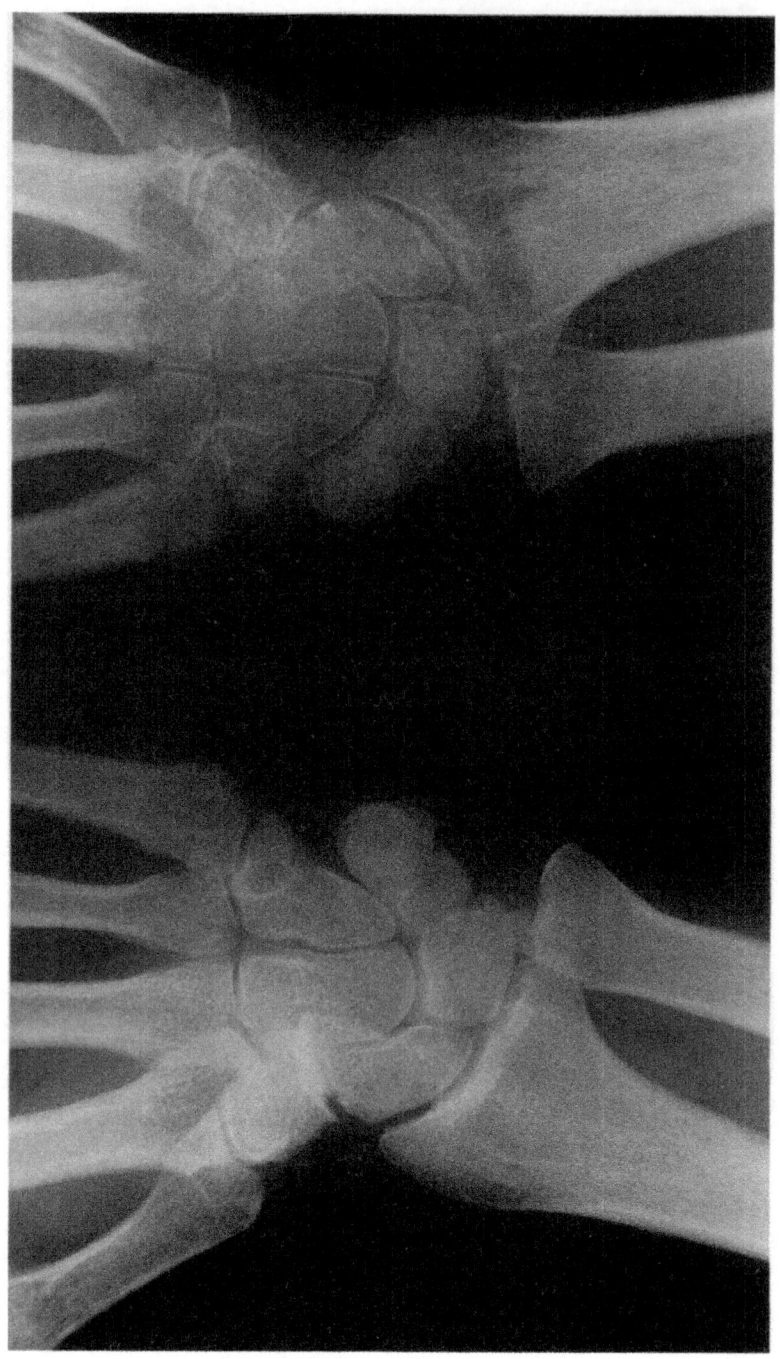

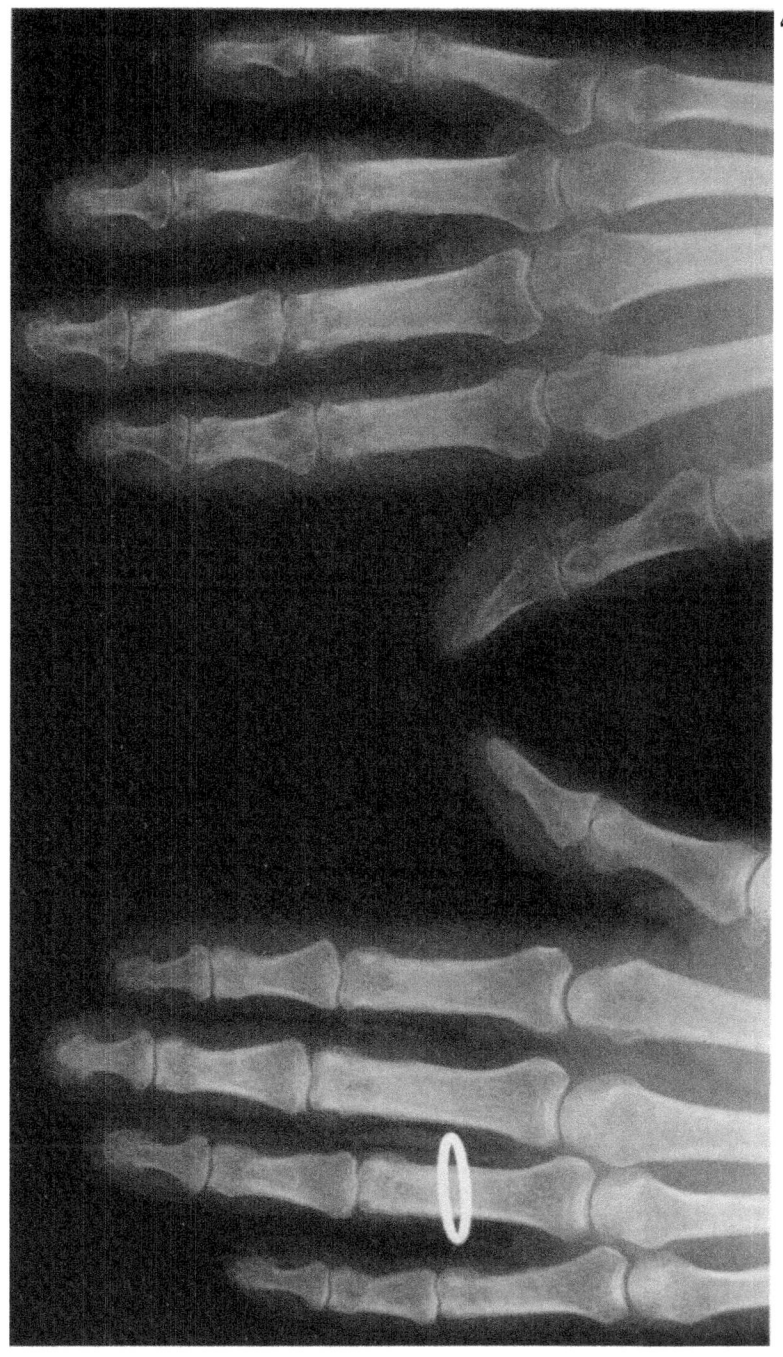

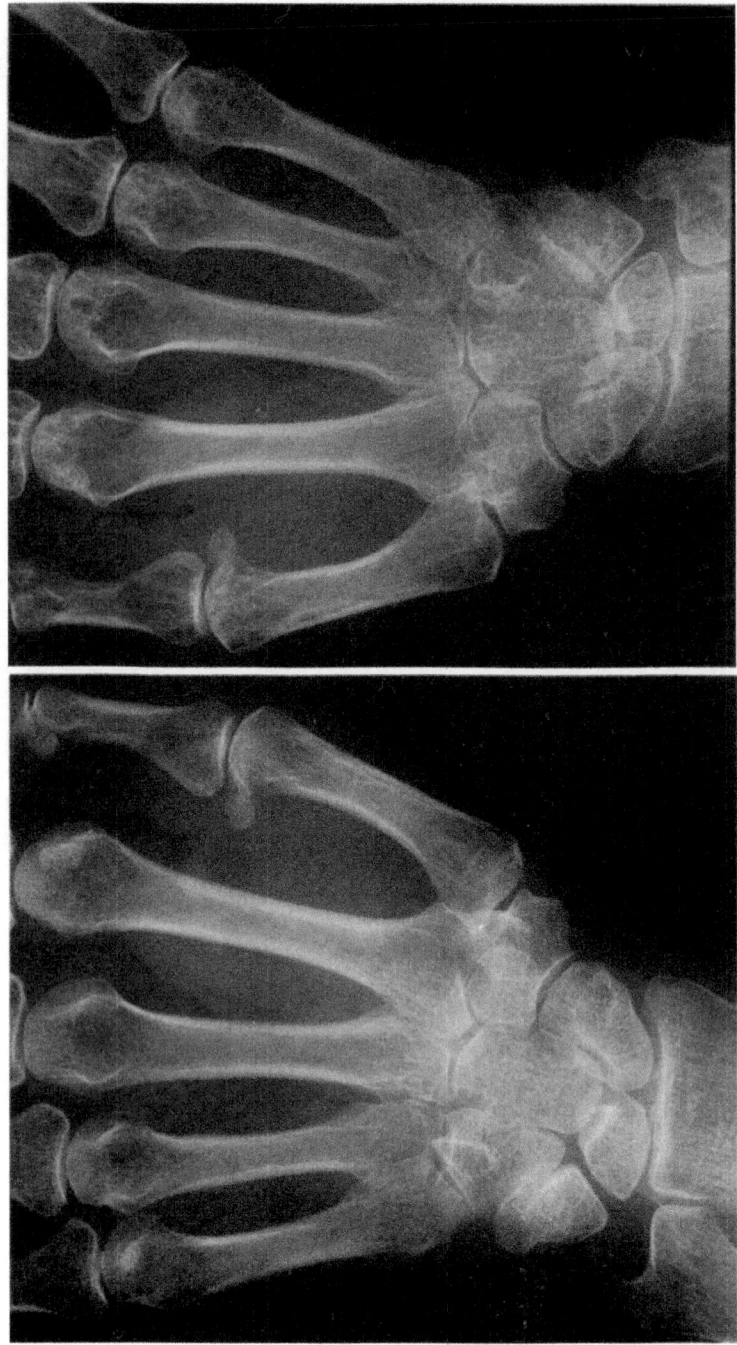

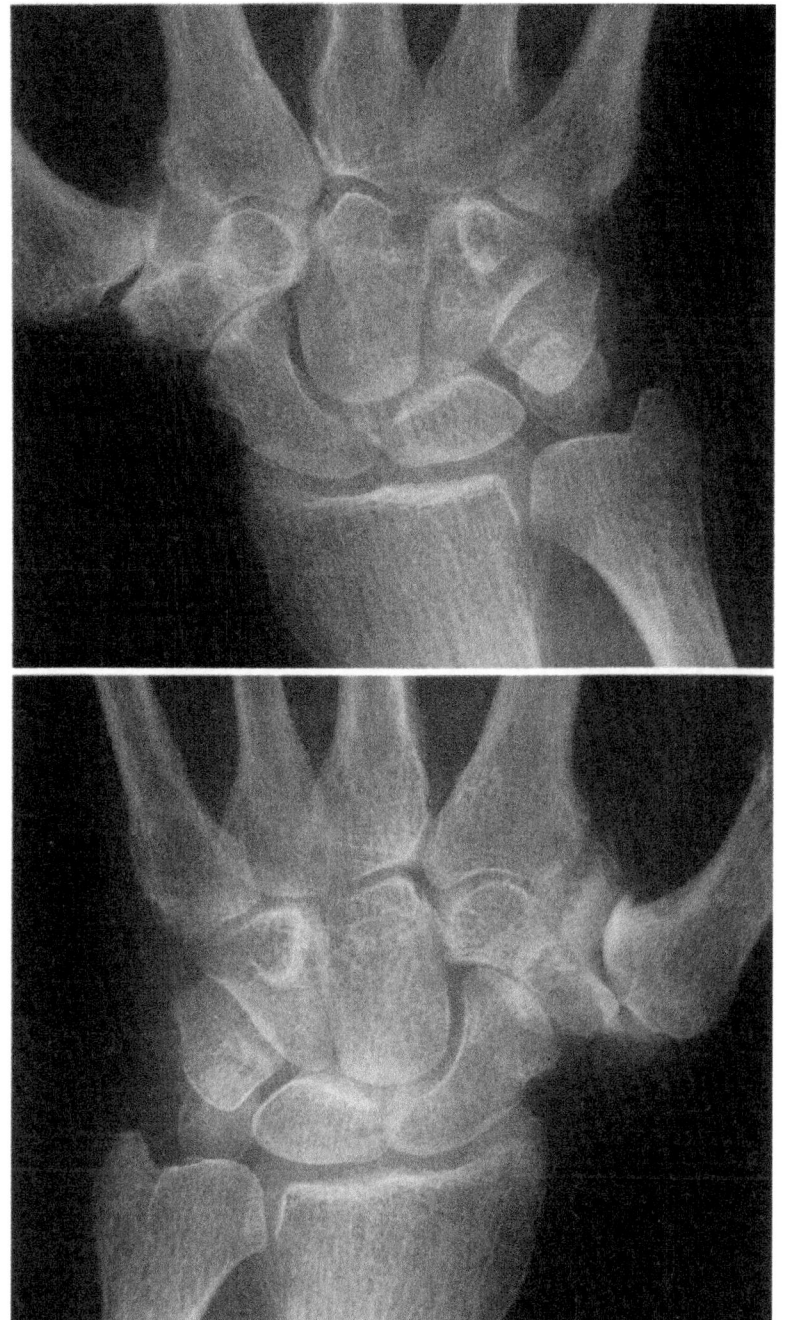

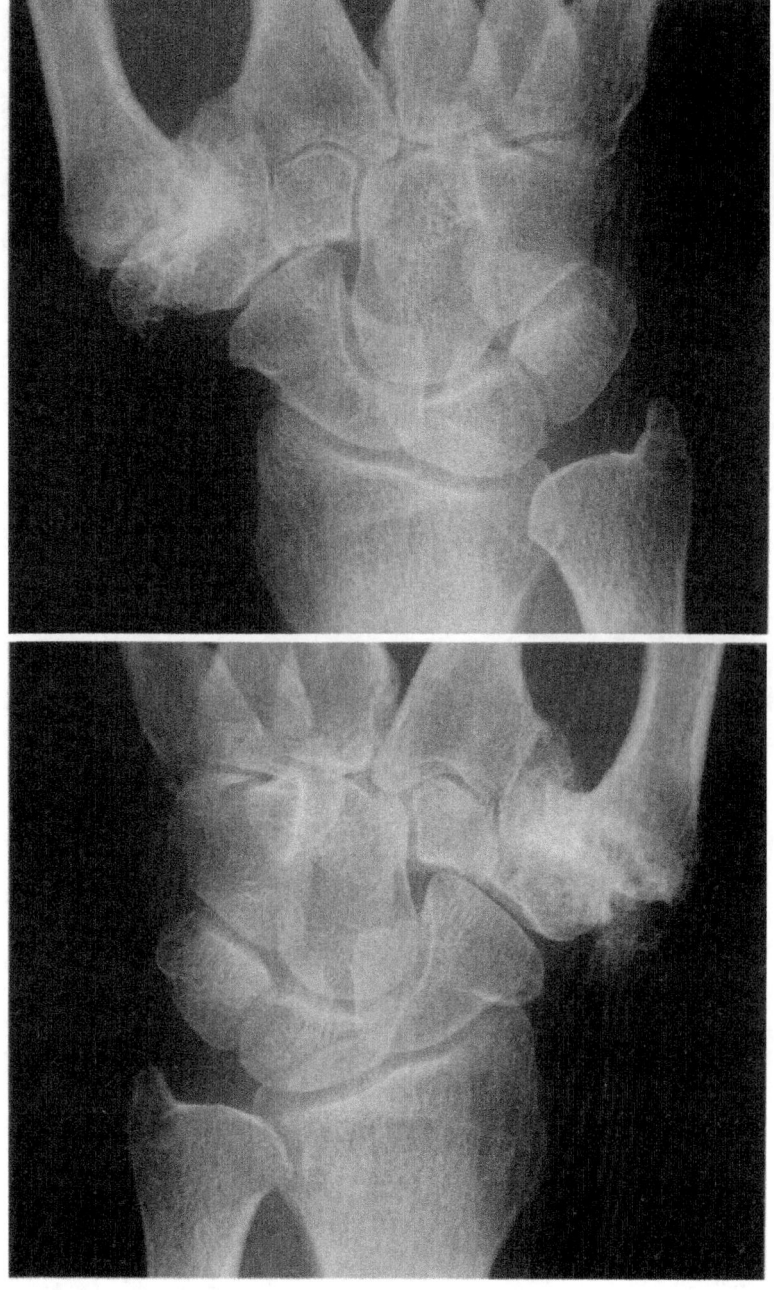

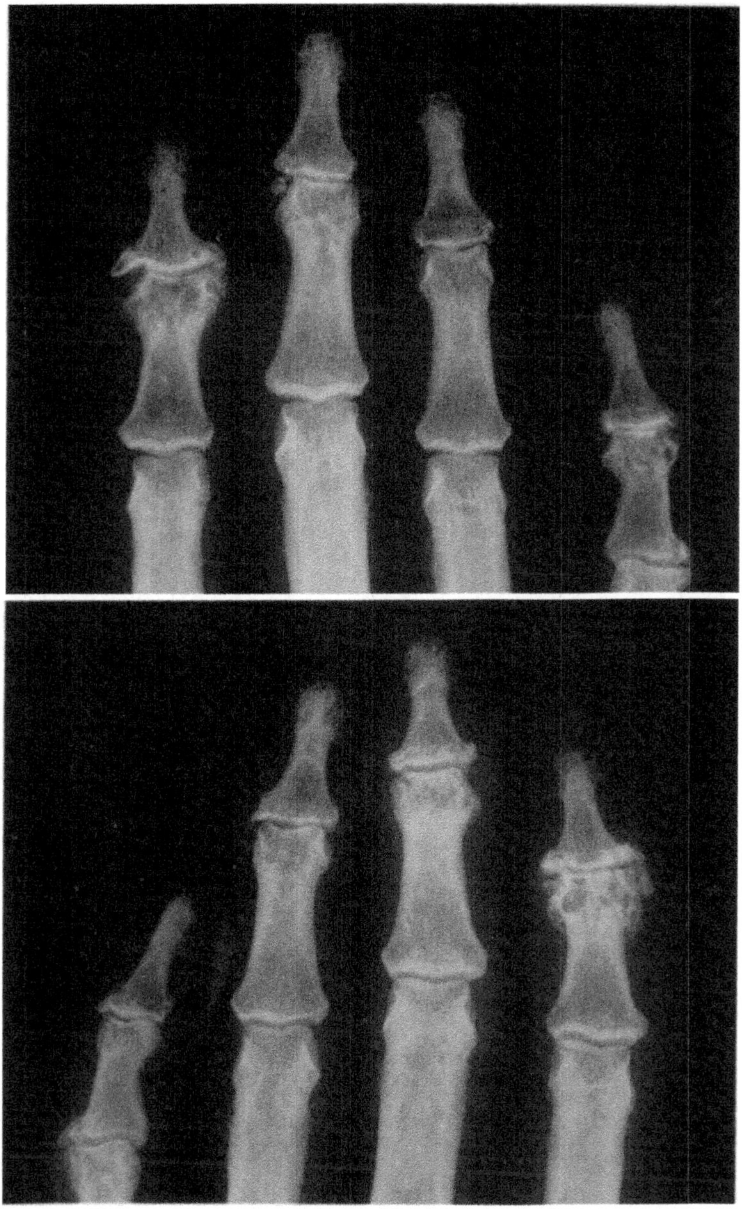

47

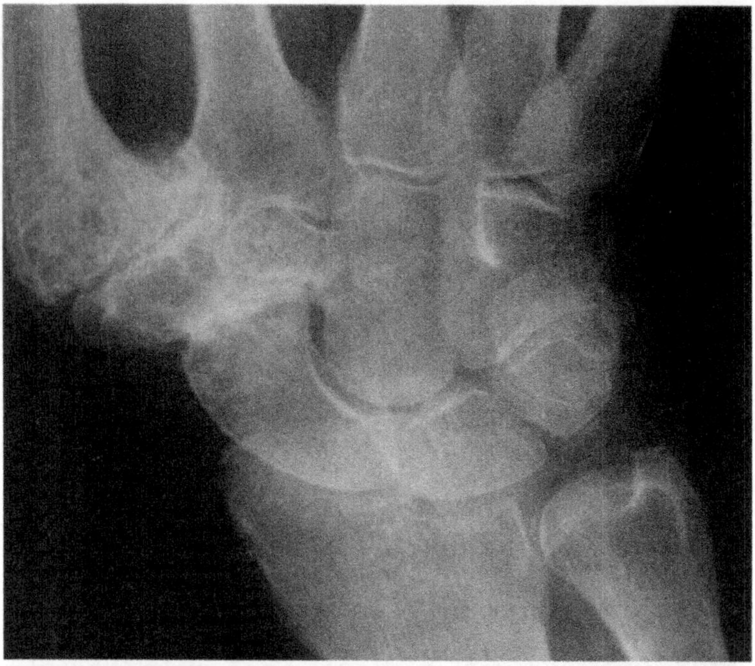

48

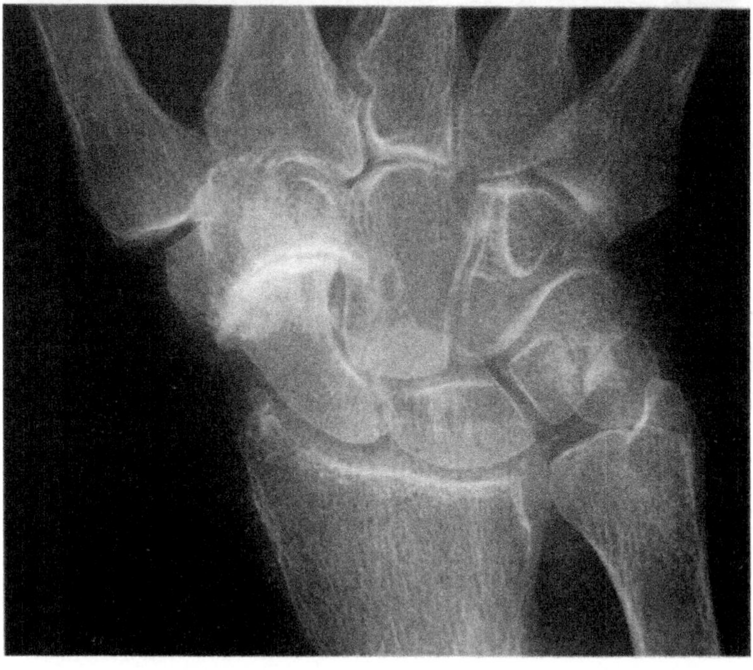

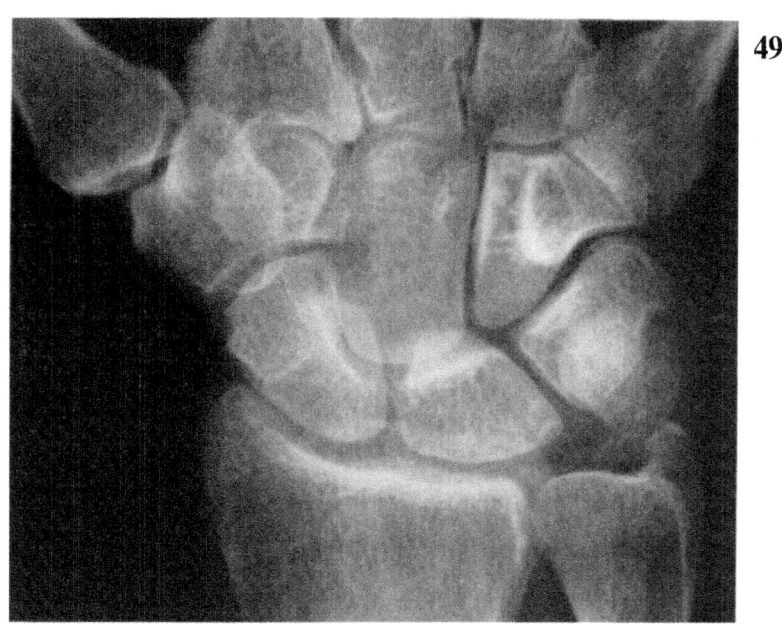

49

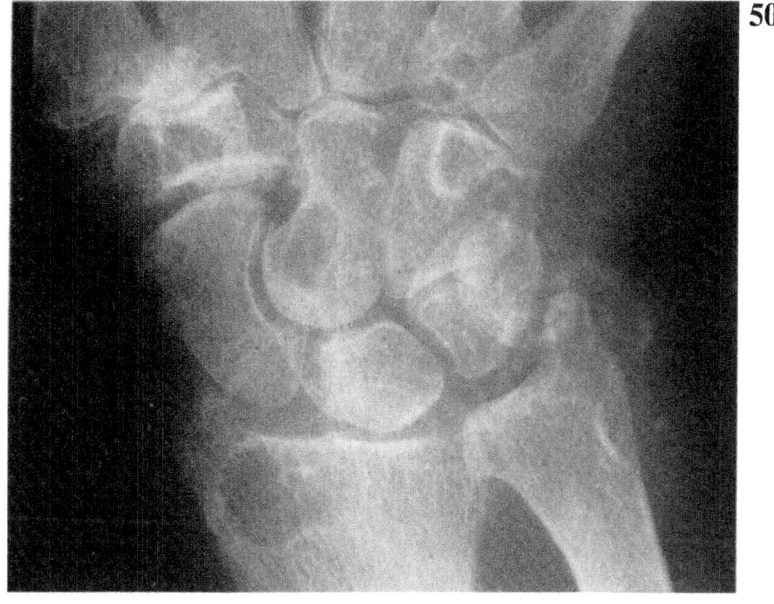

50

51

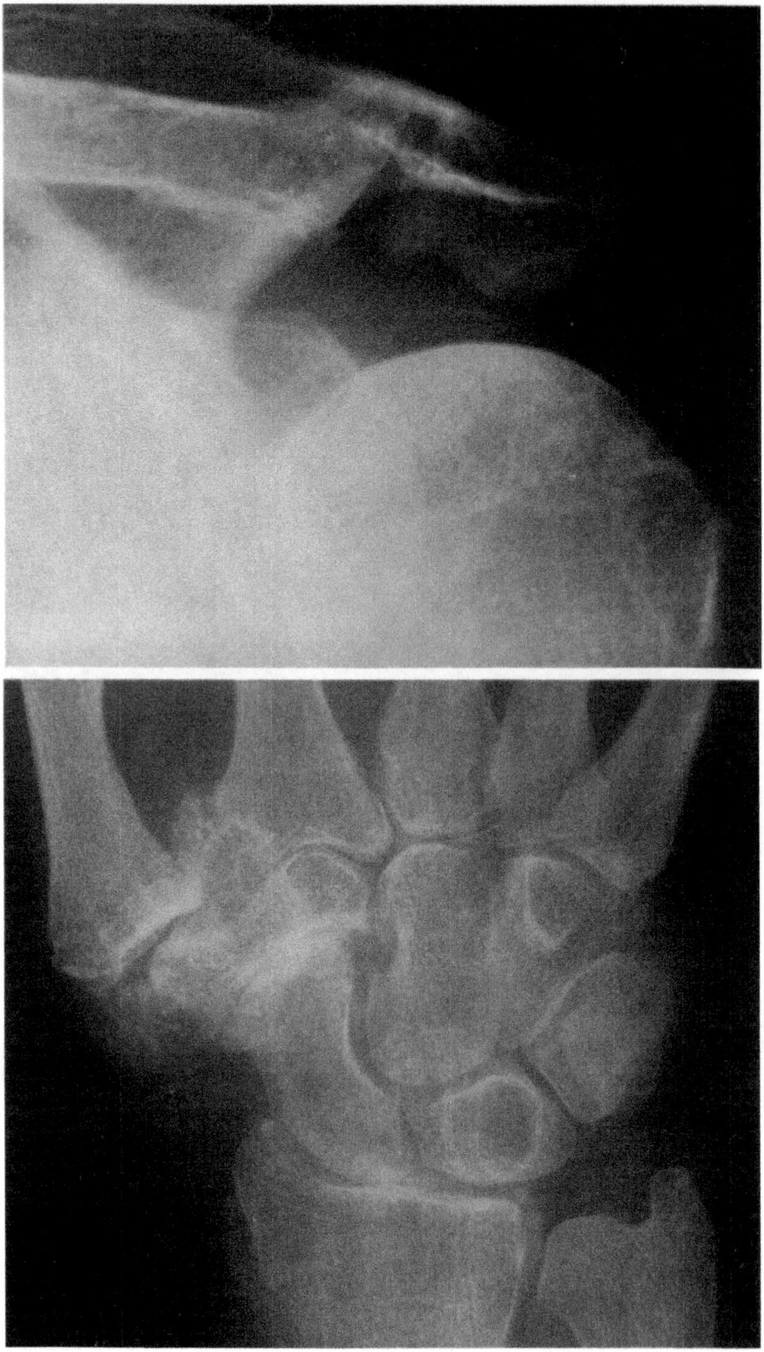

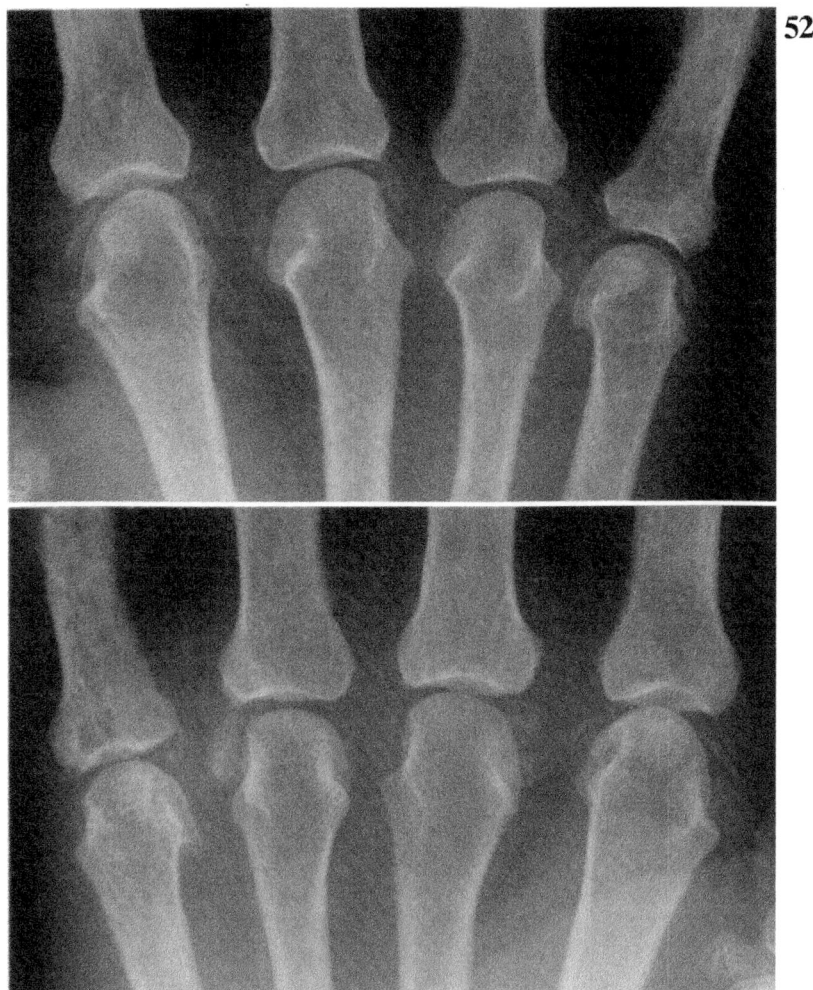

53

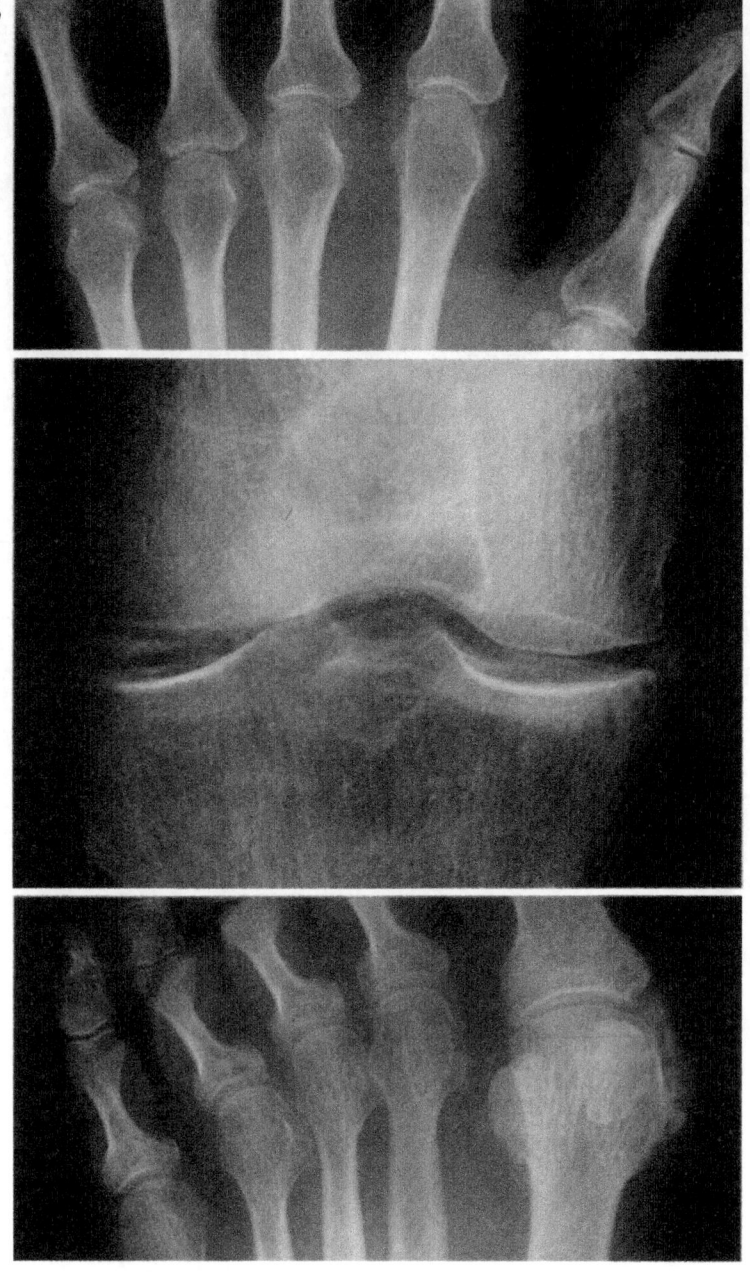

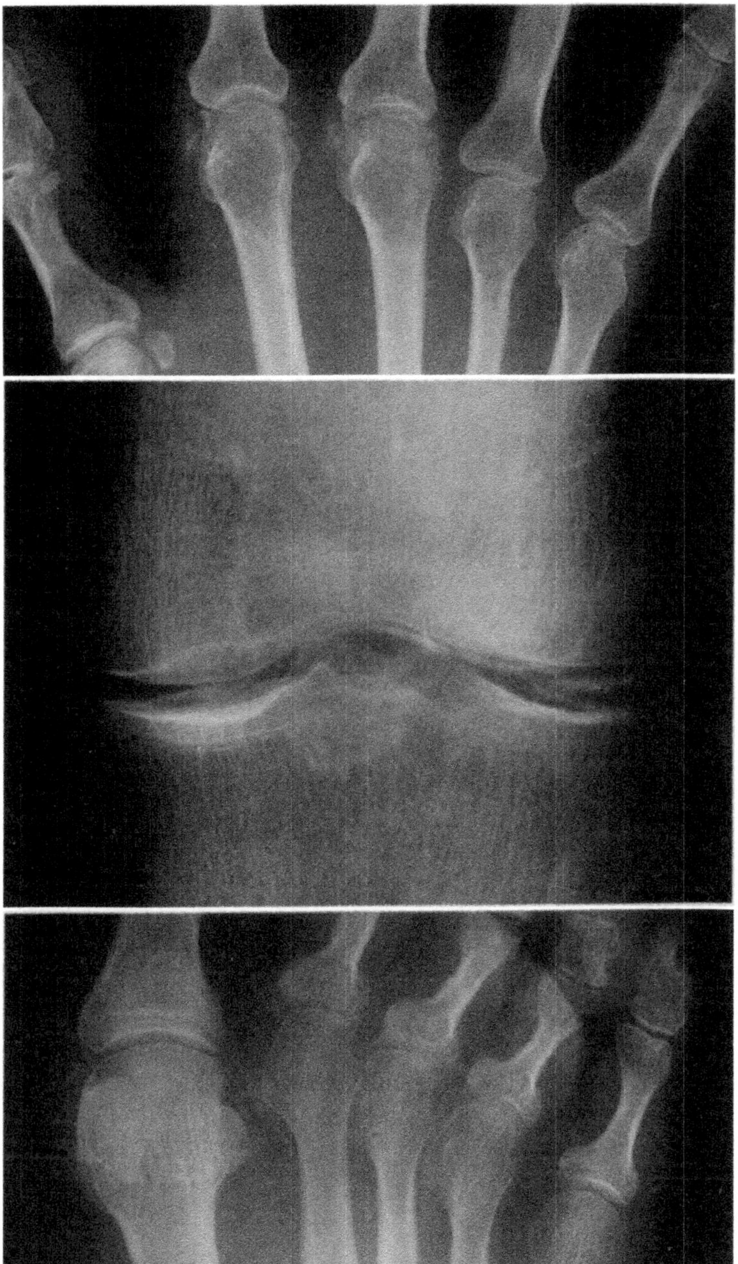

54

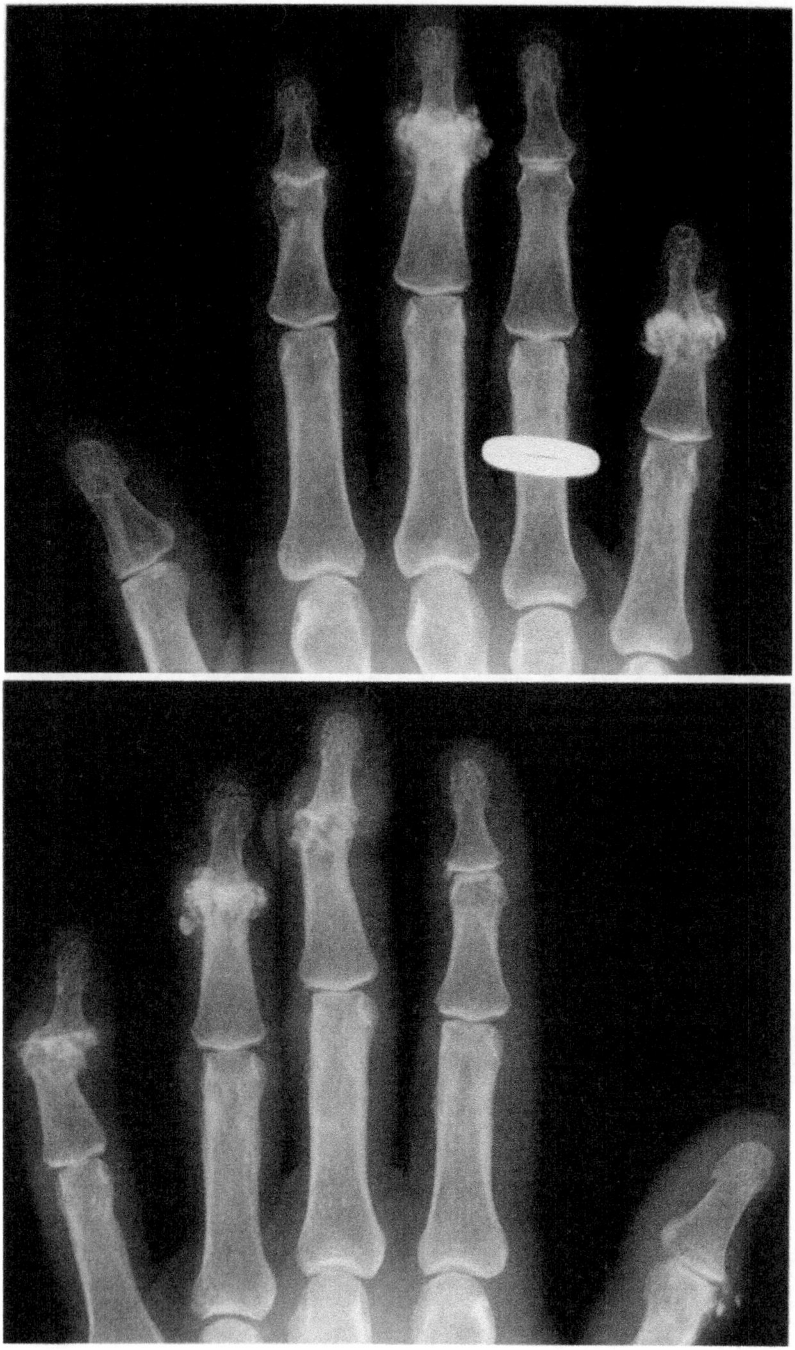

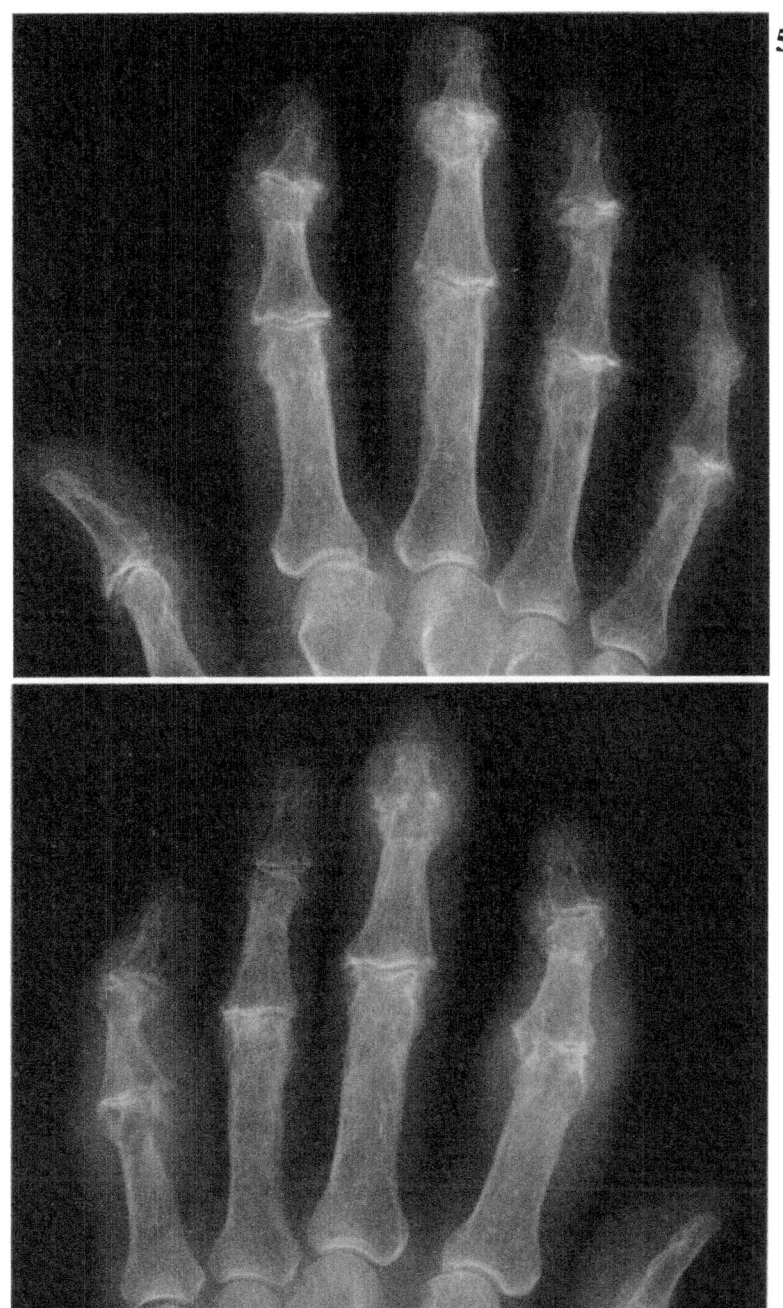

55

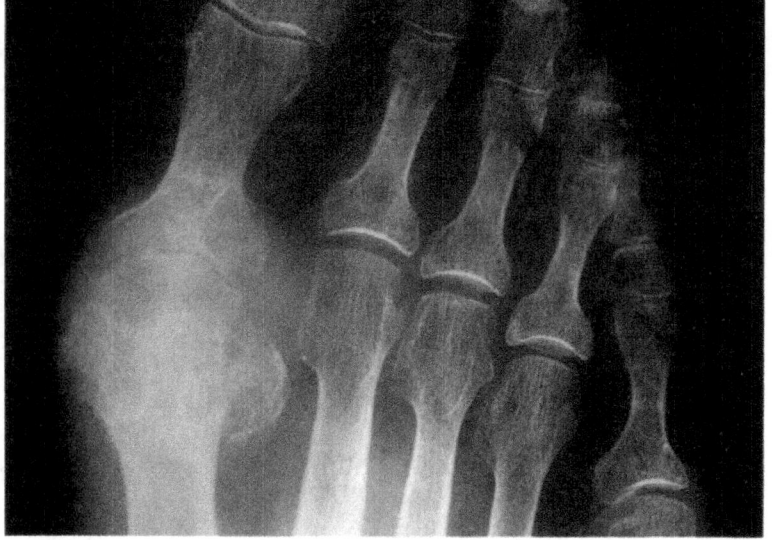

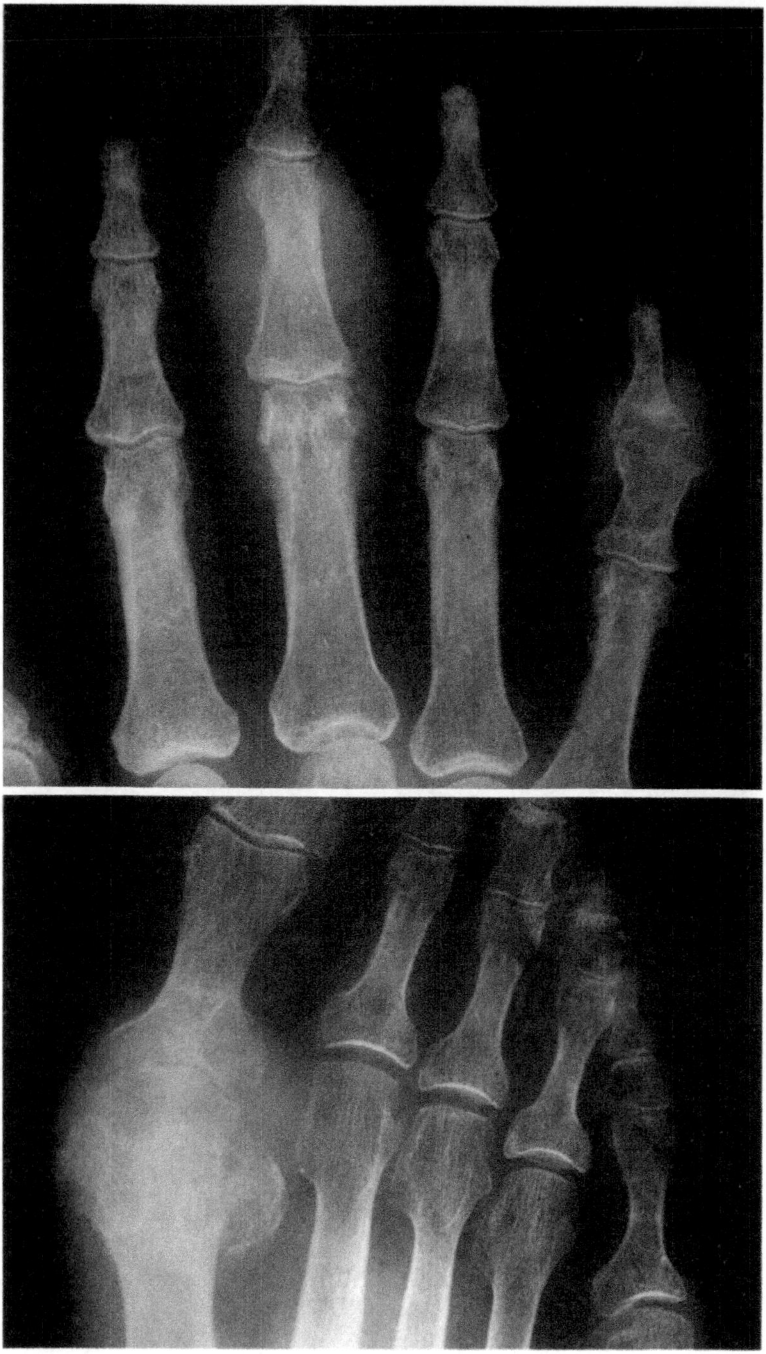

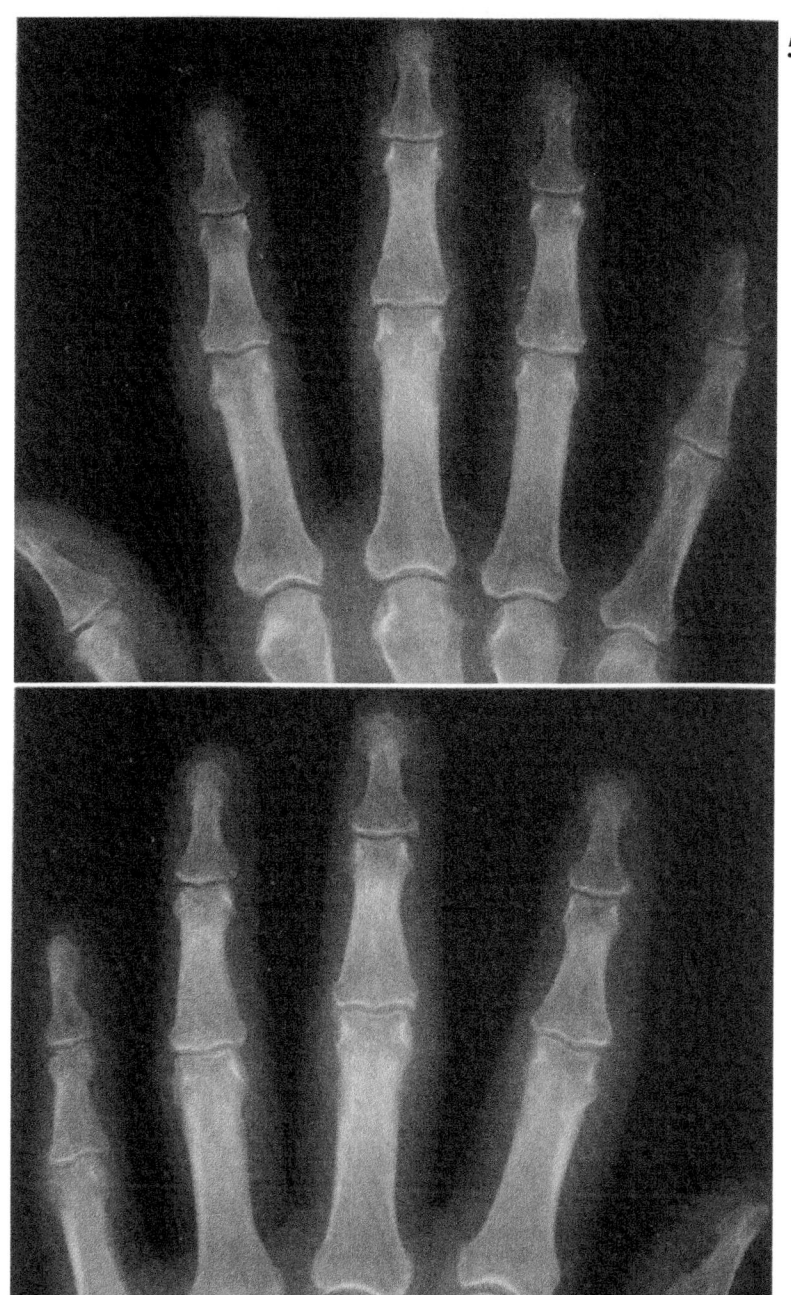

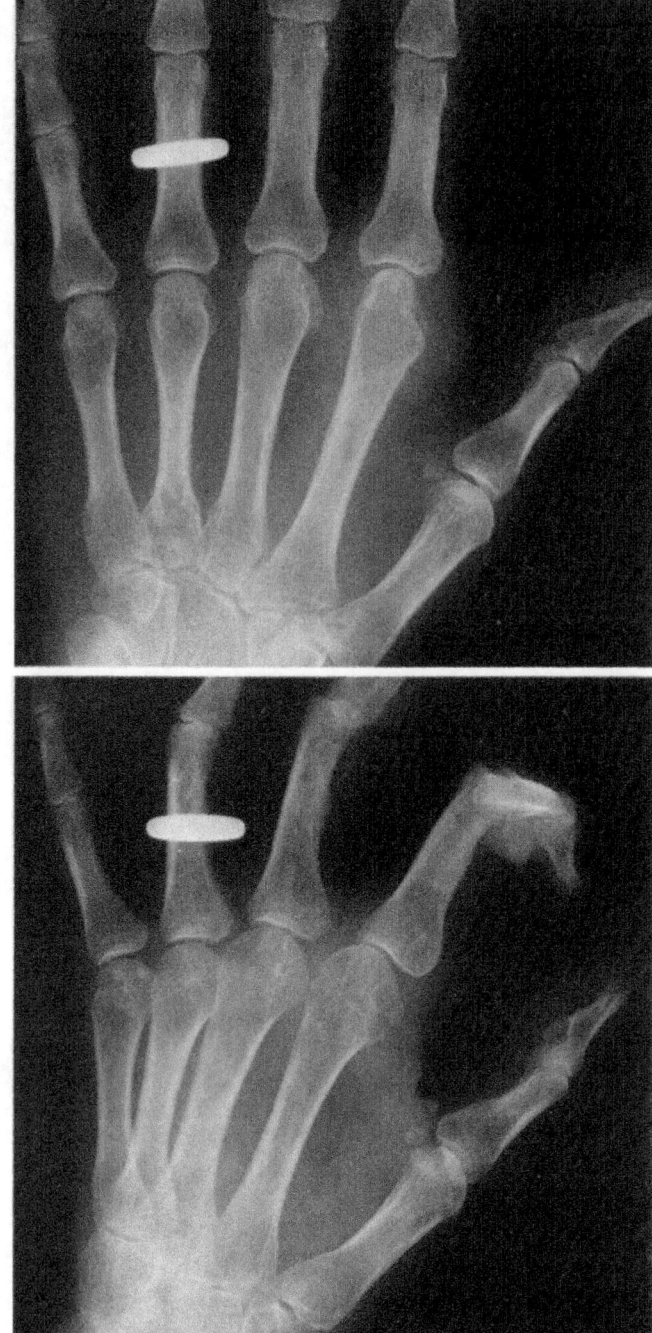

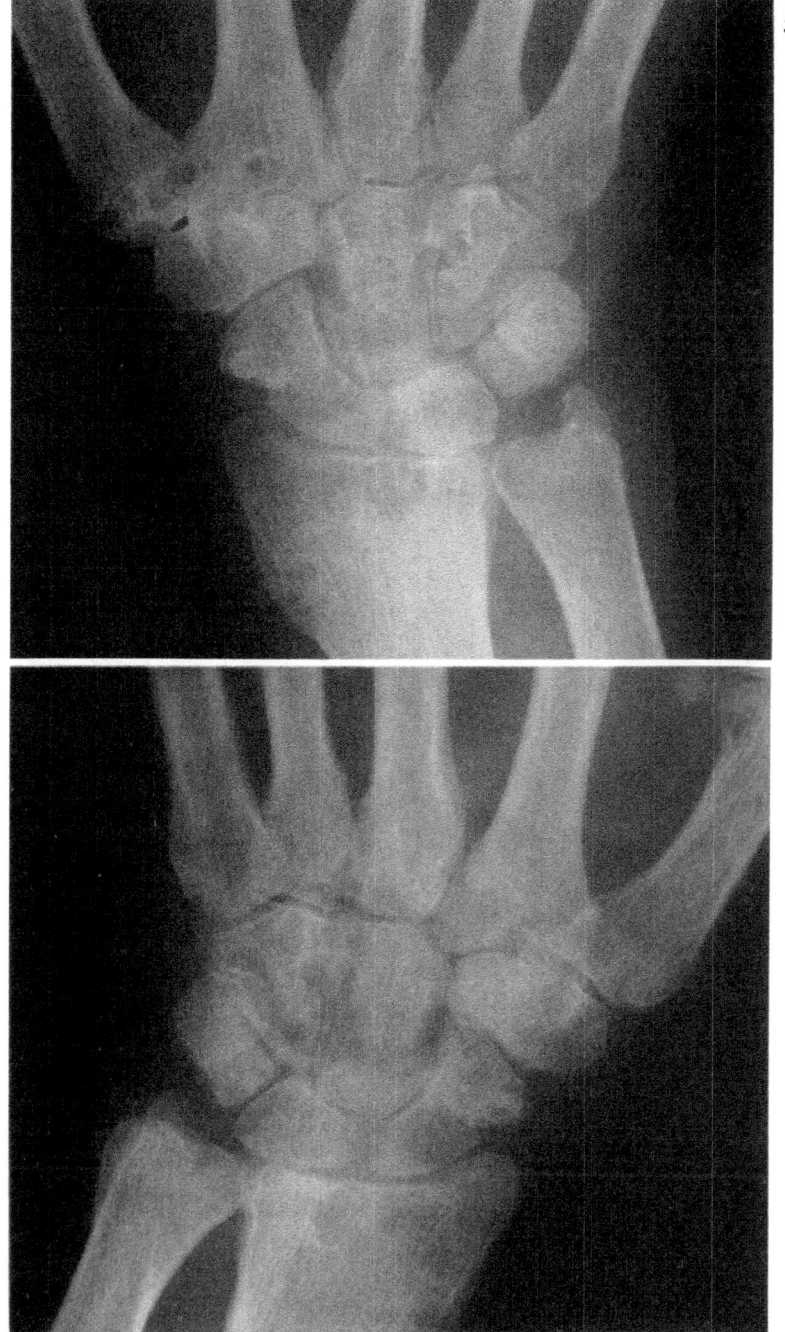

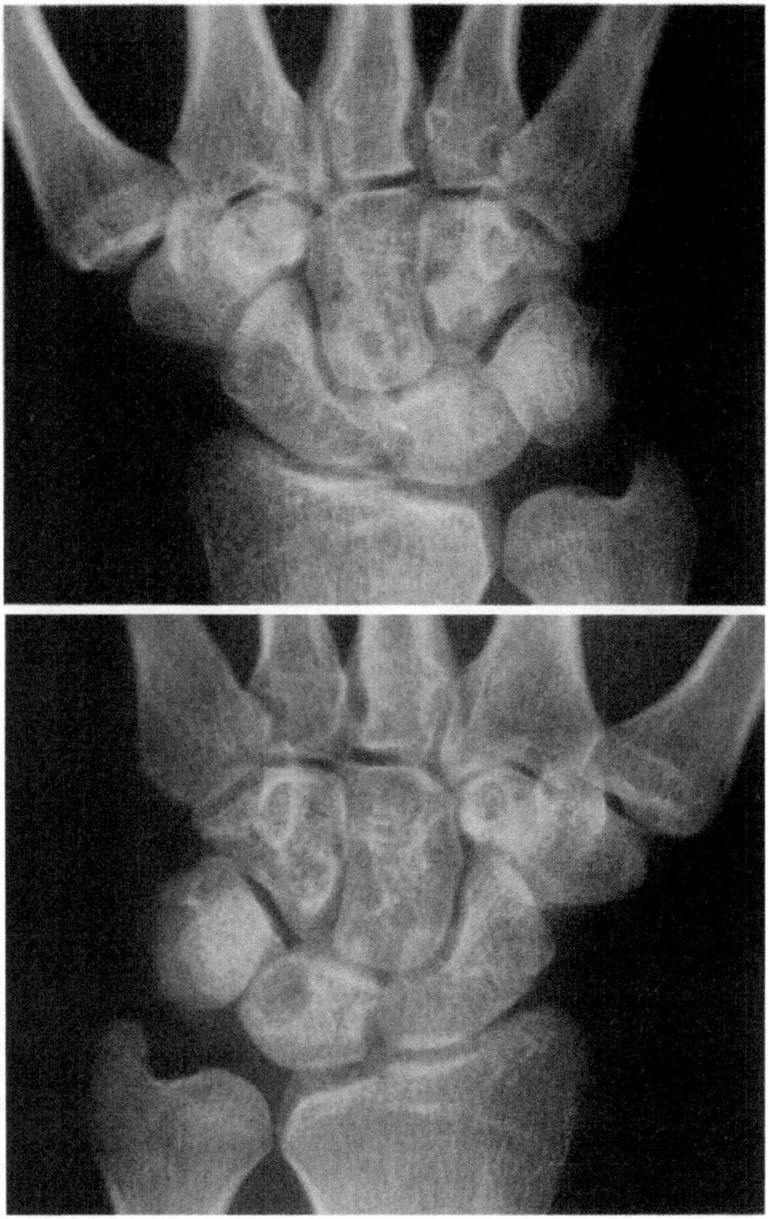

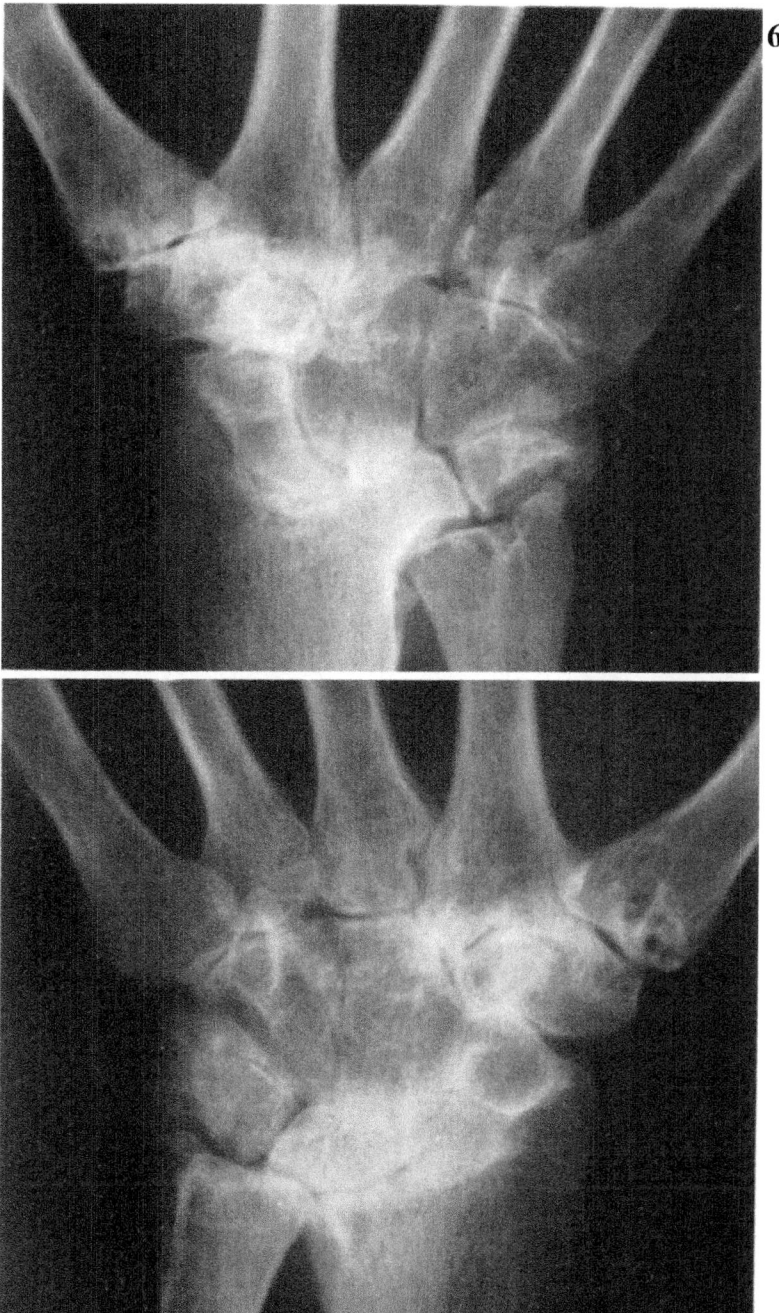

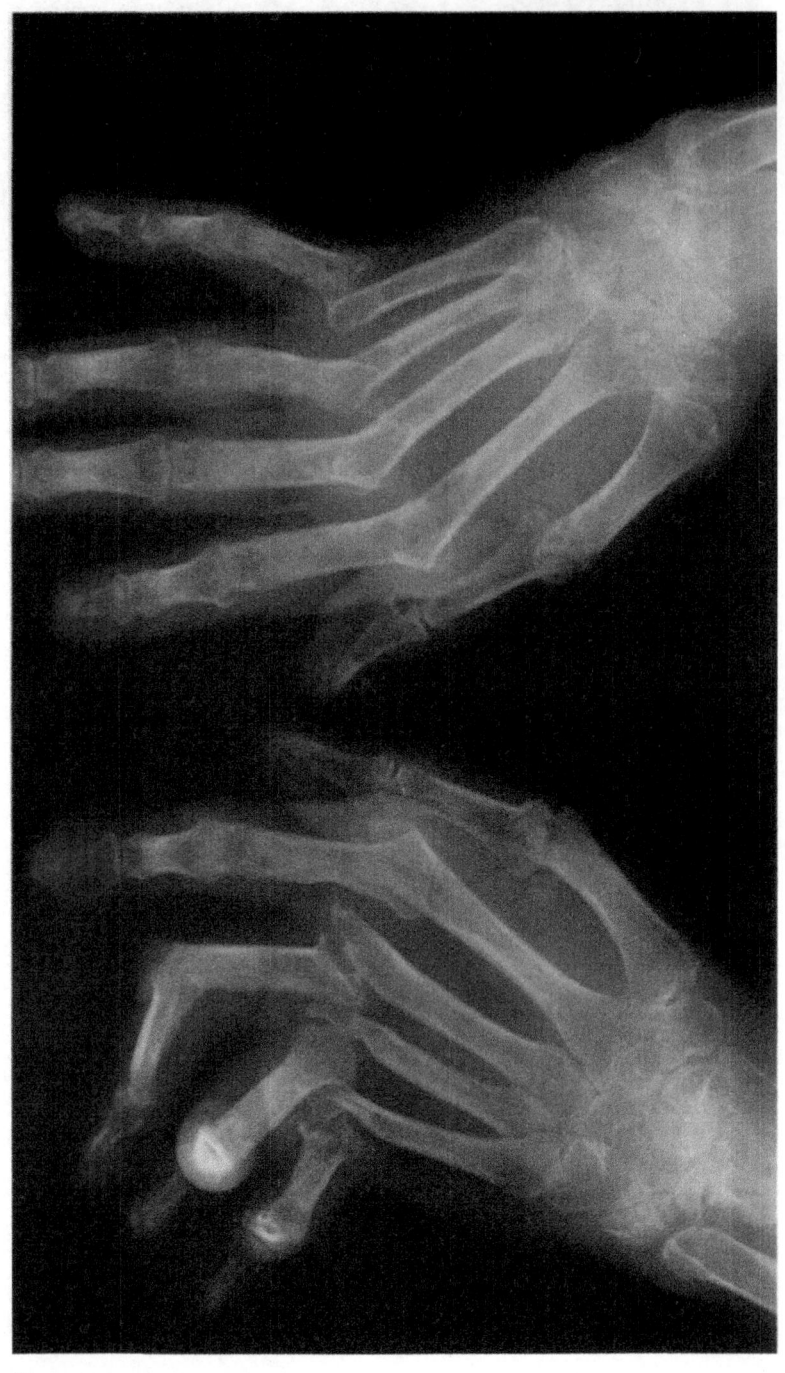

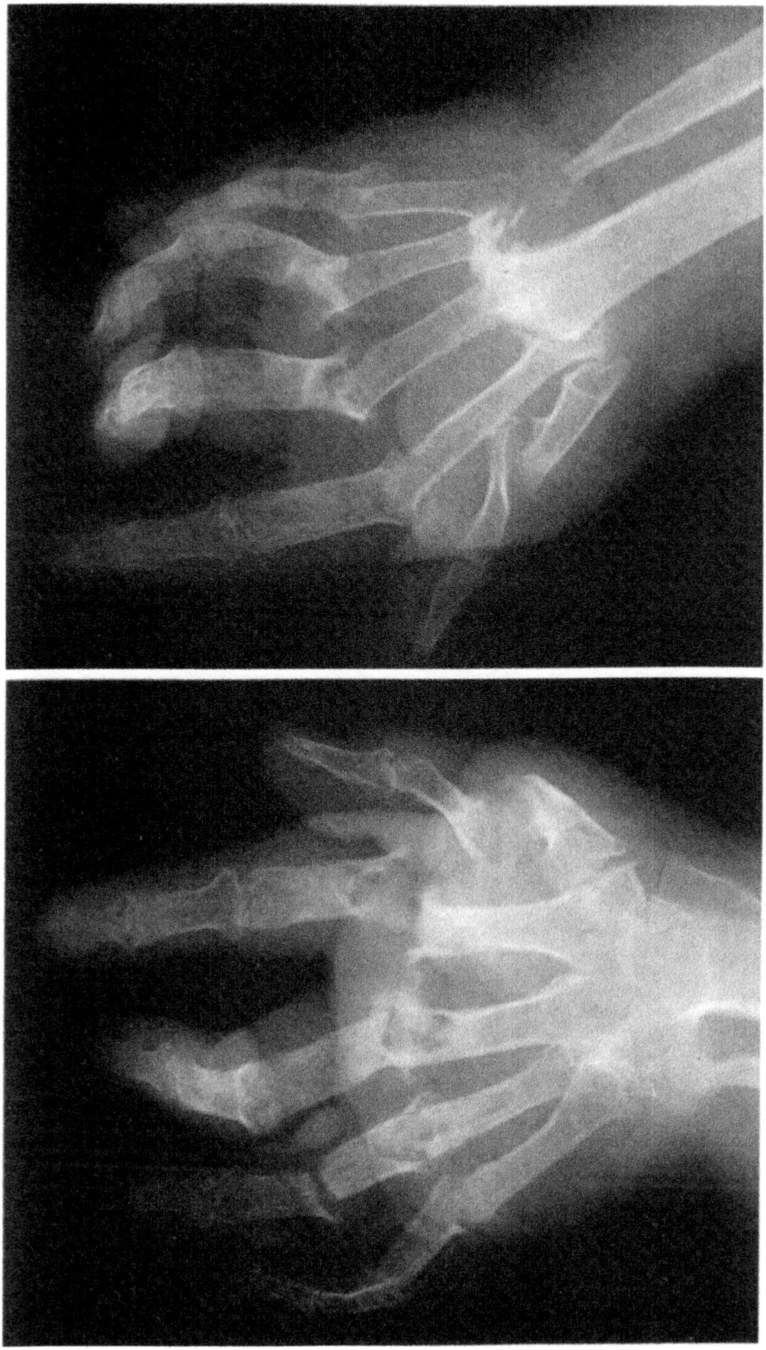

64

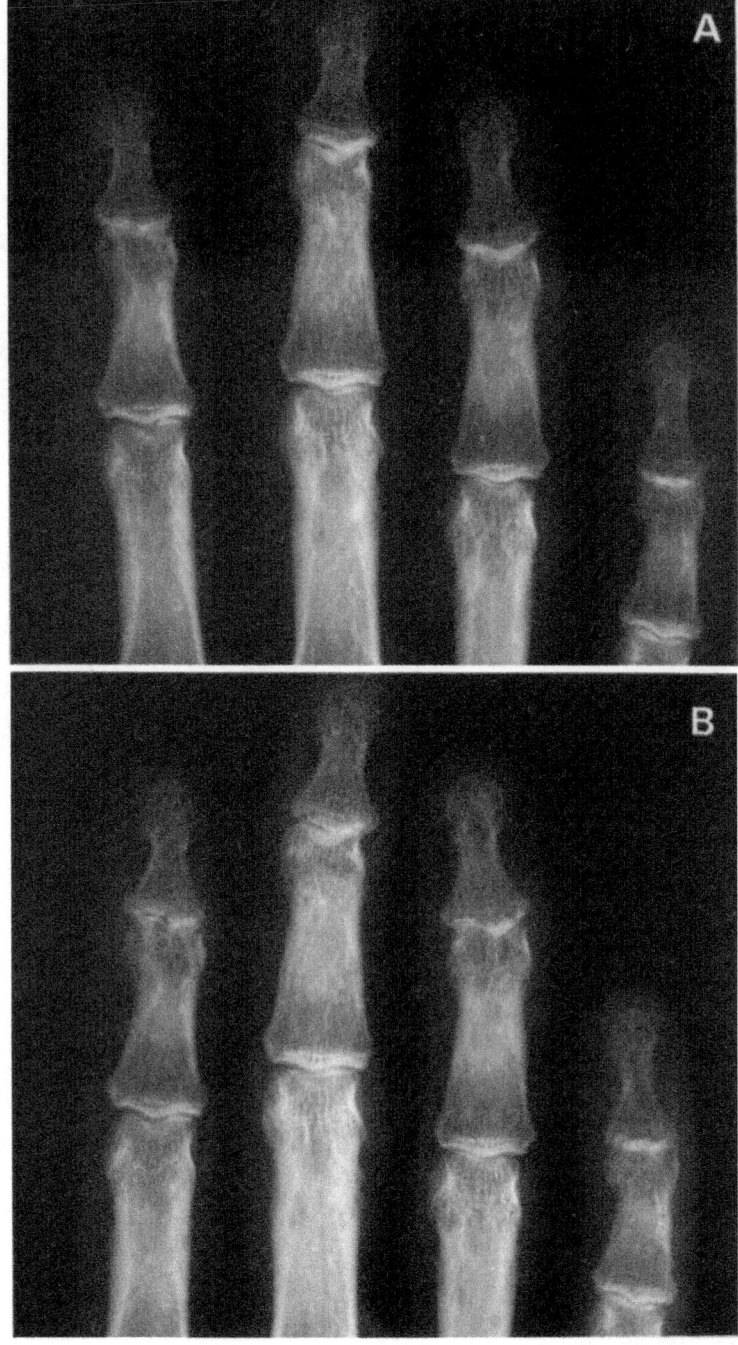

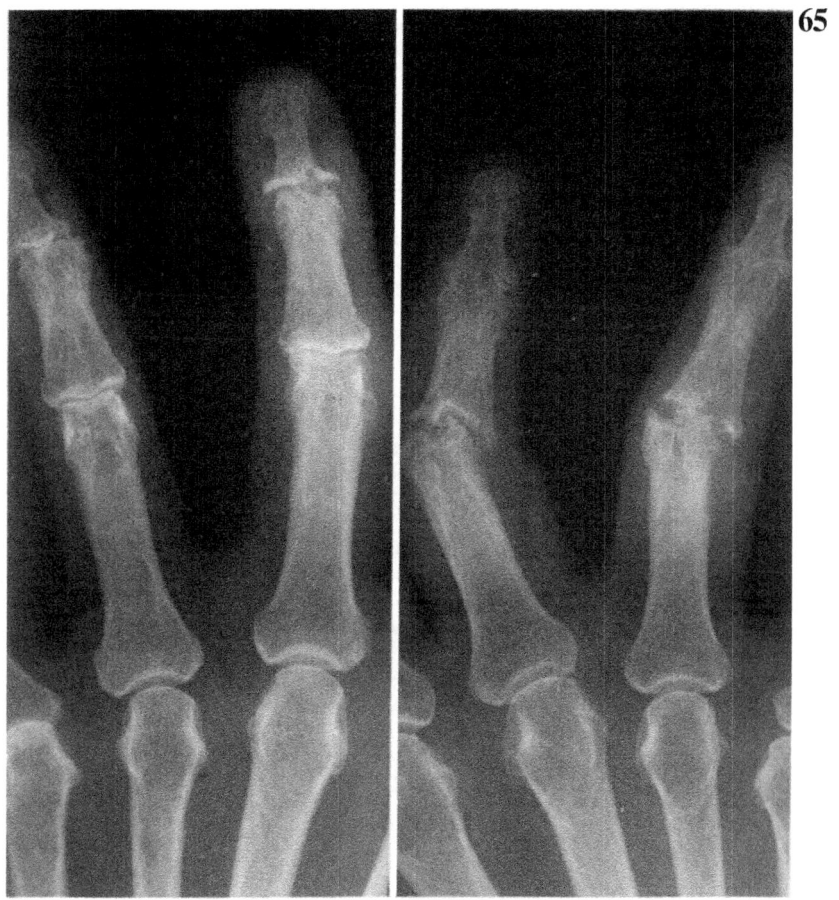

66

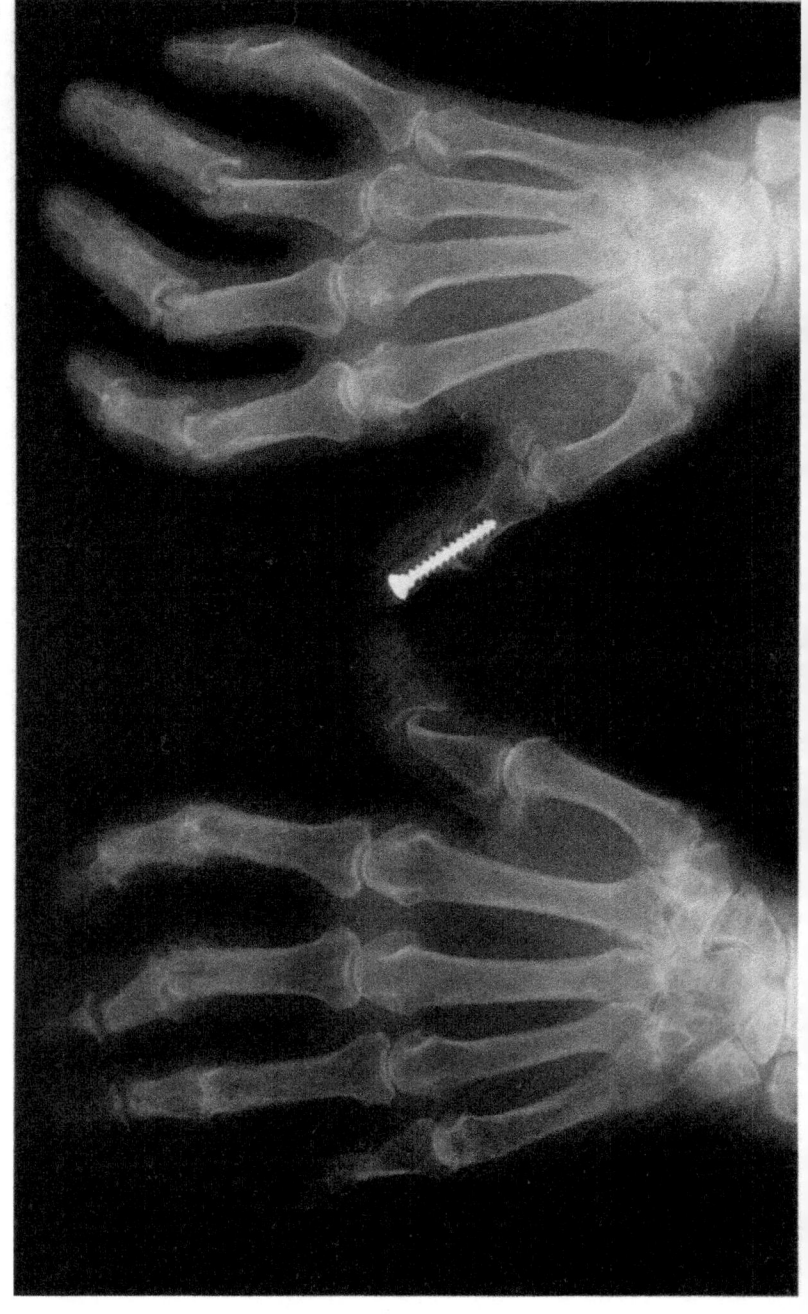

48

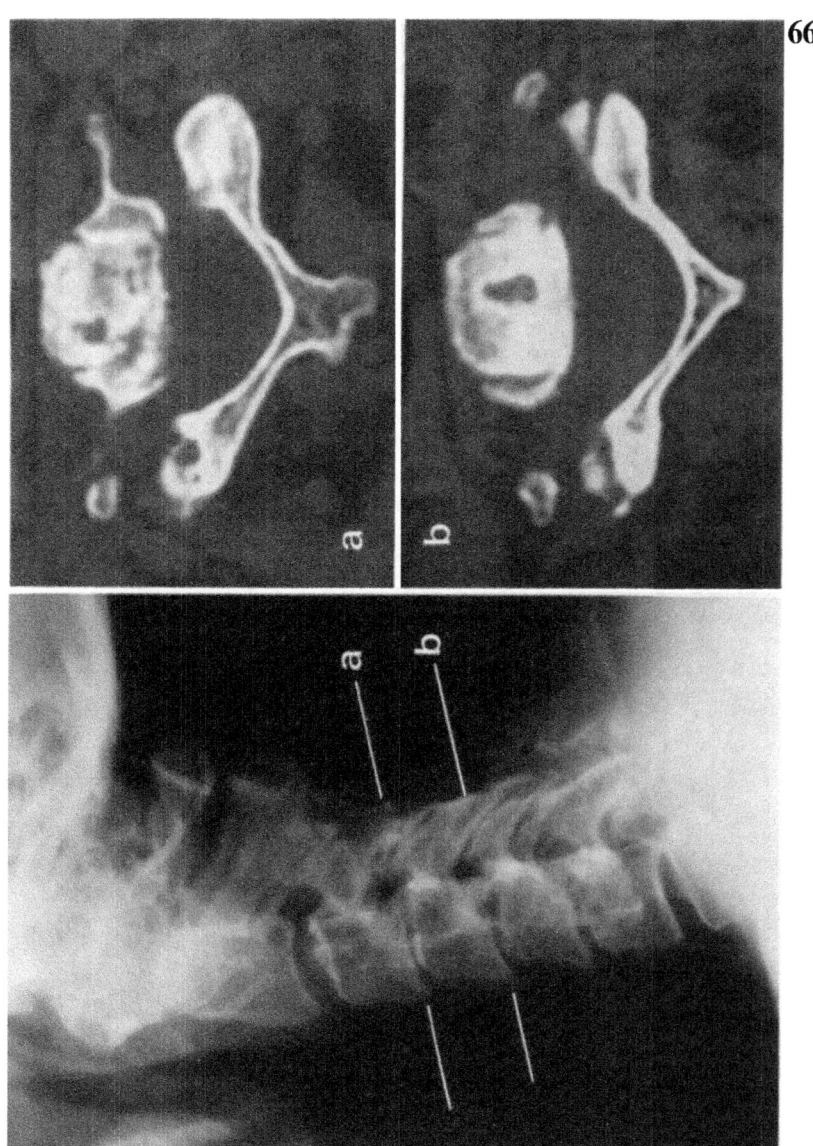

66

67

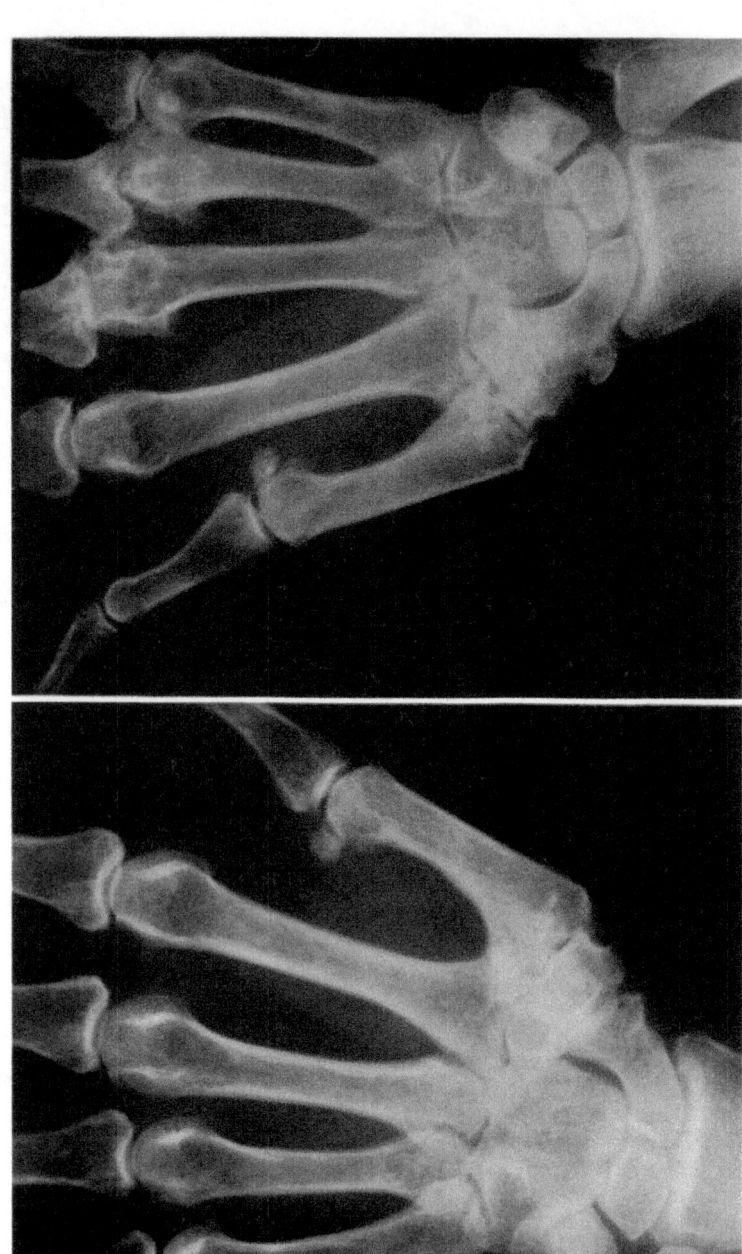

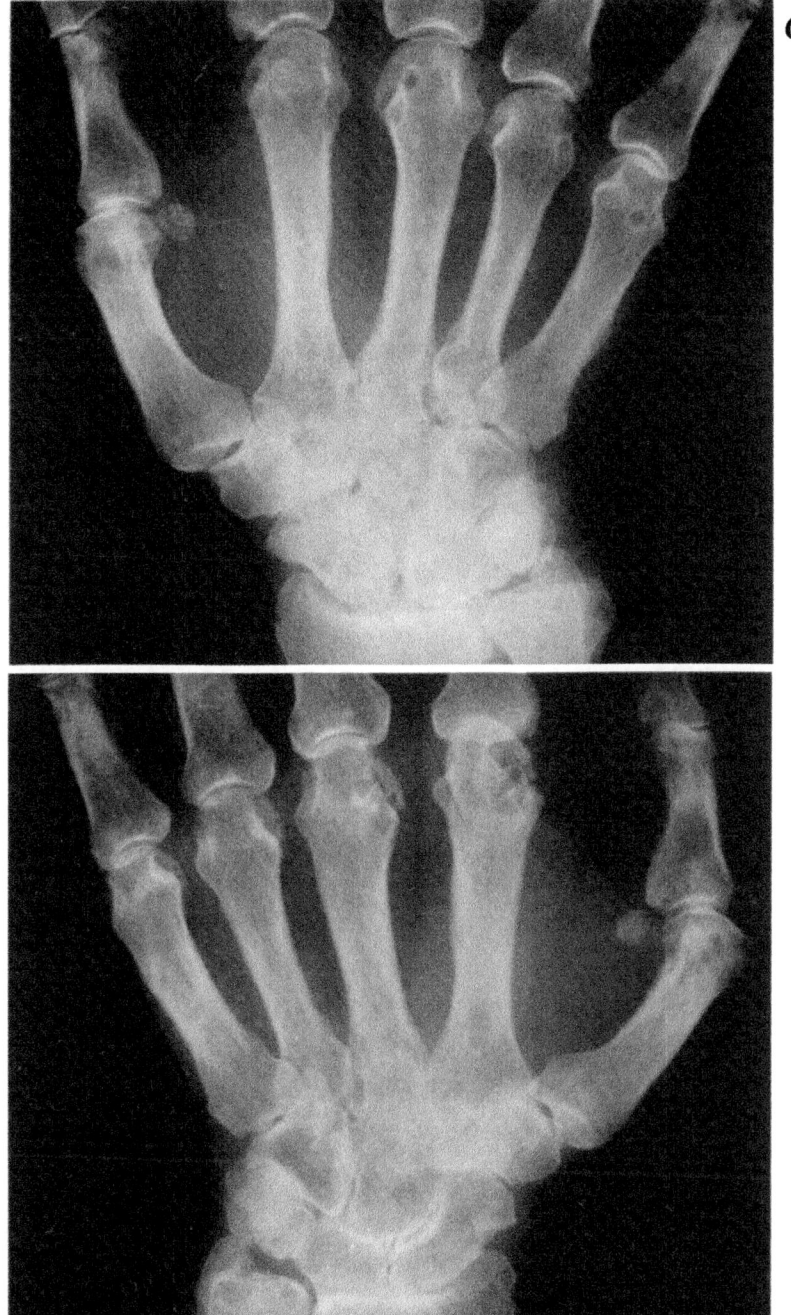

69

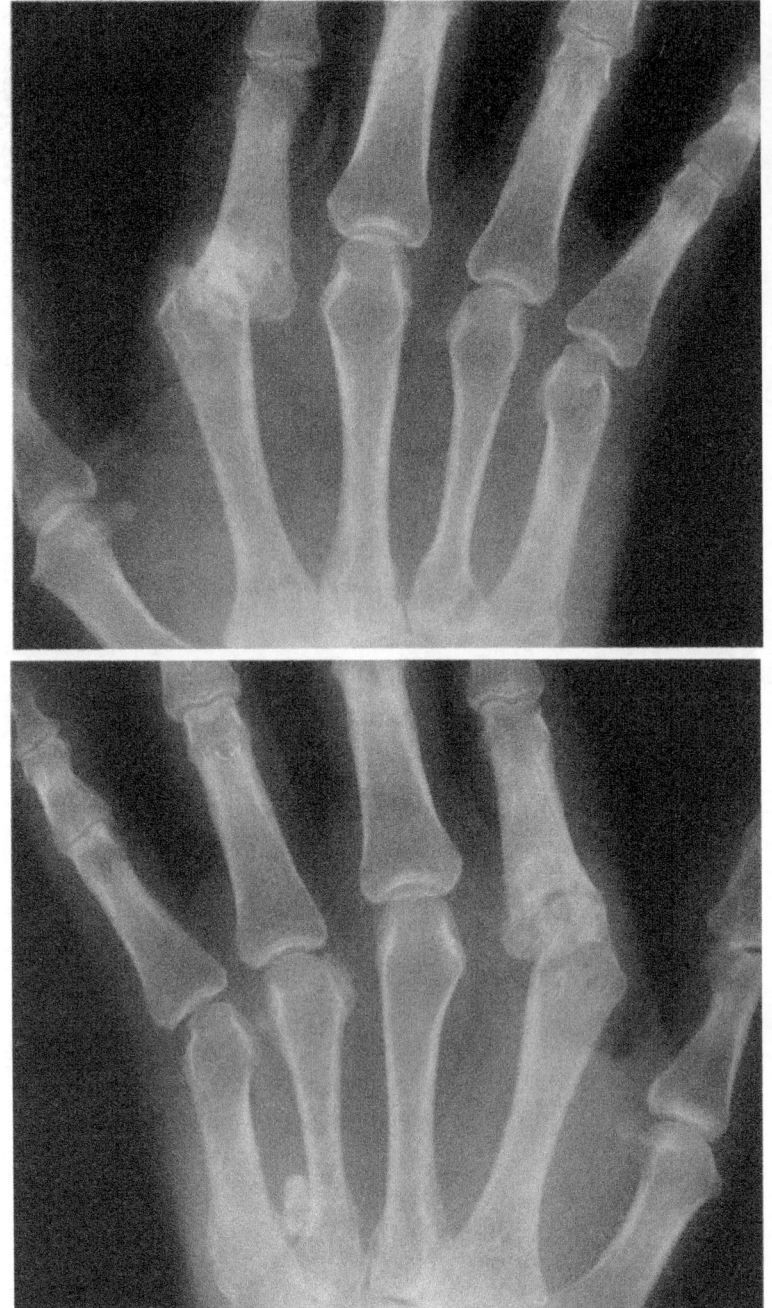

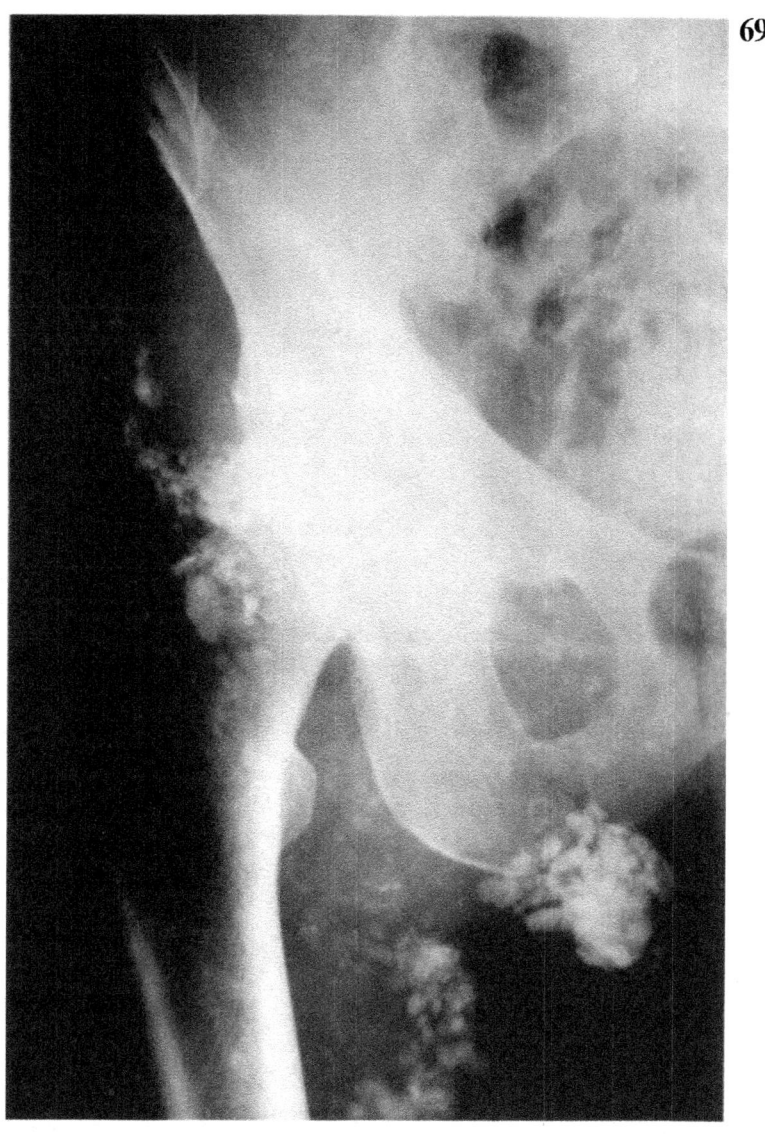

70

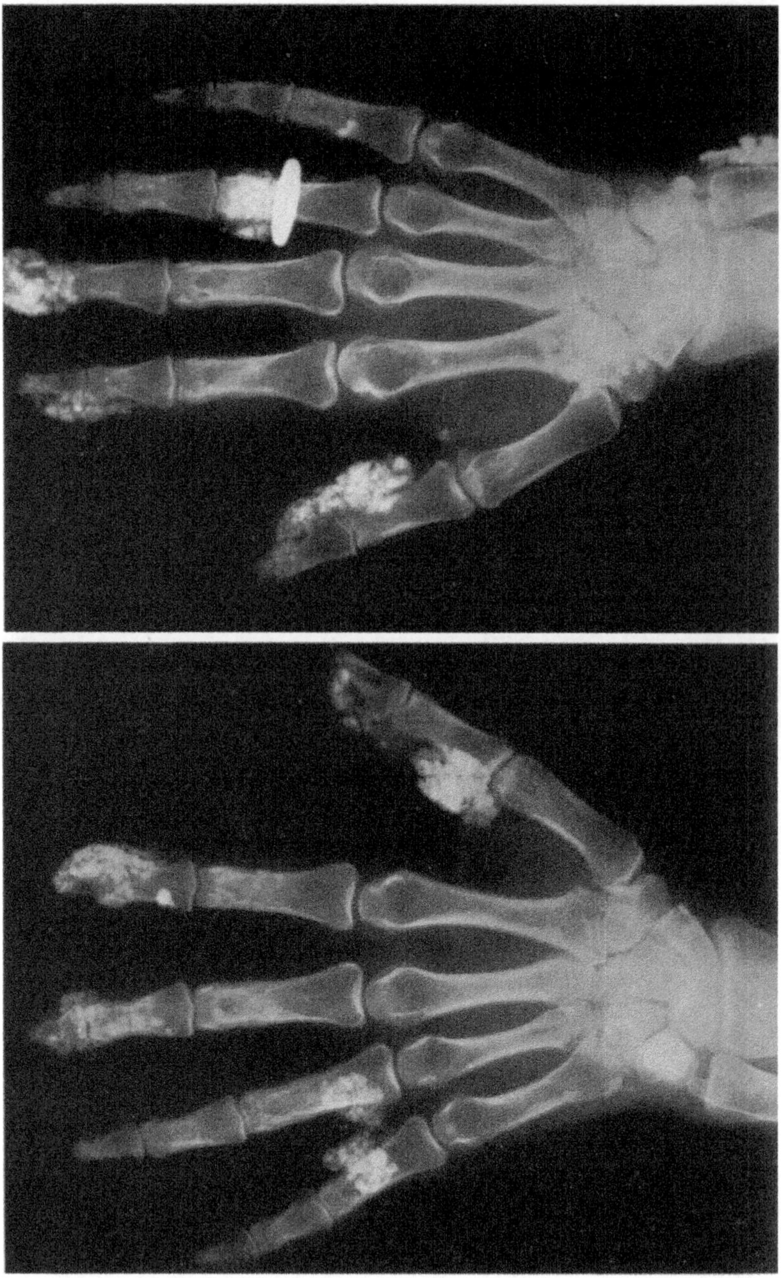

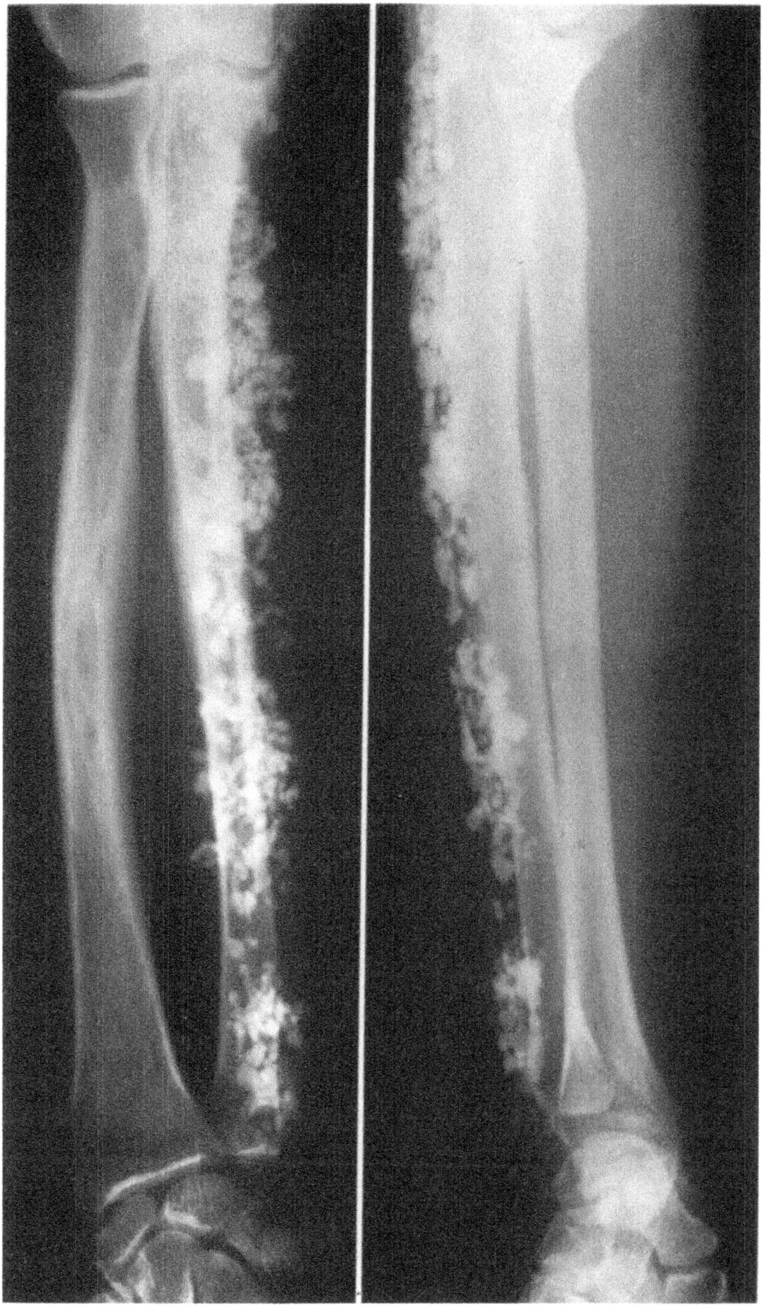

71

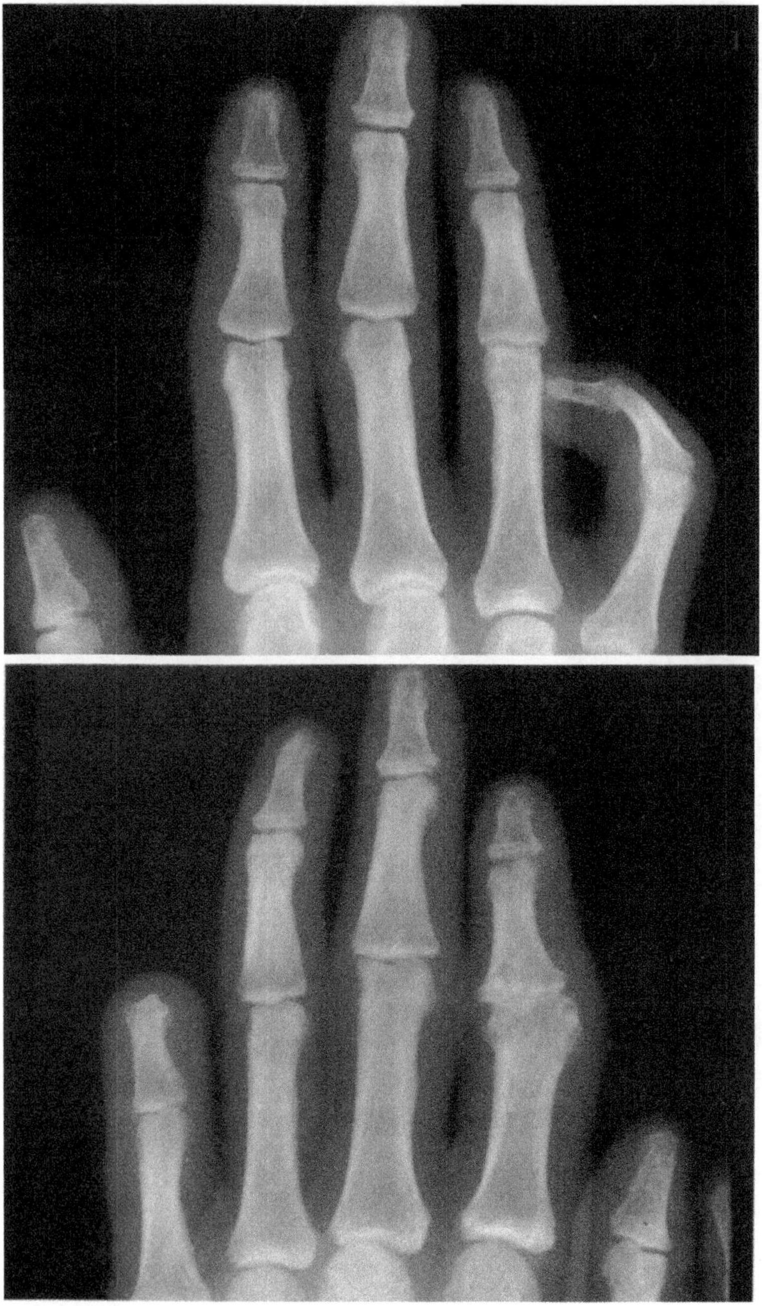

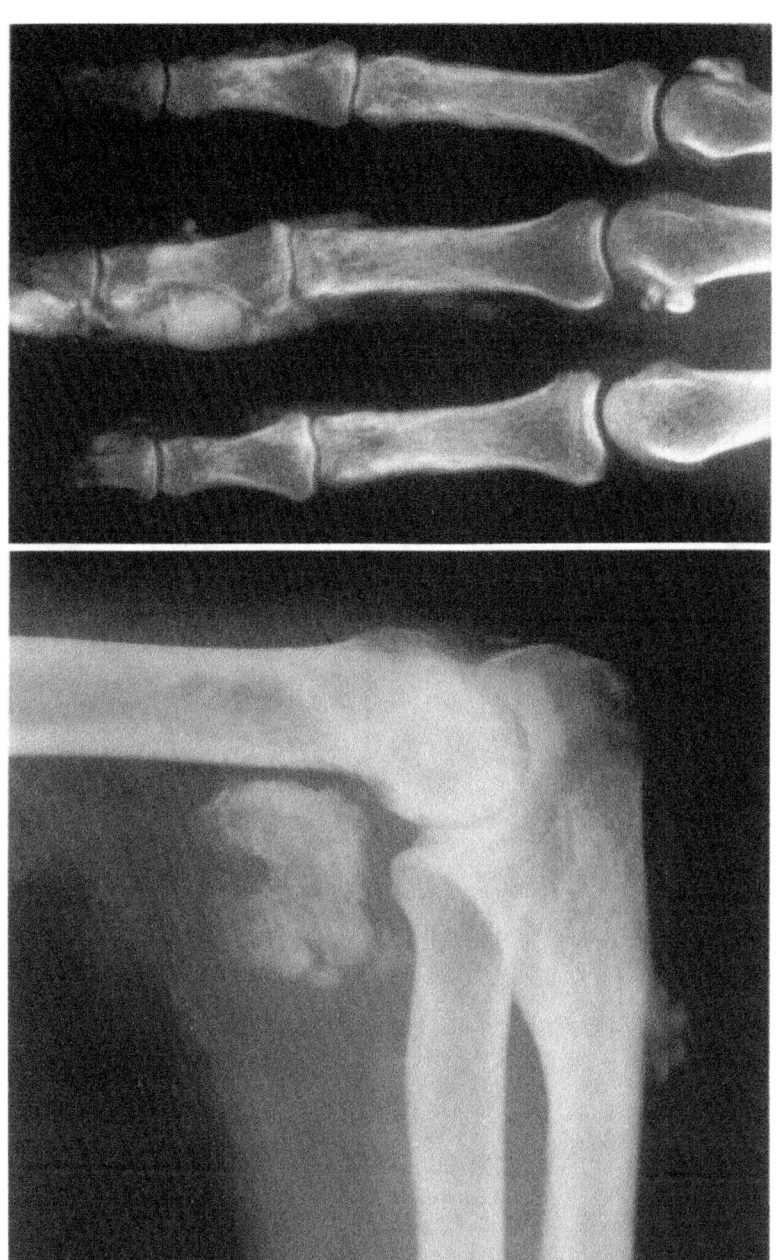

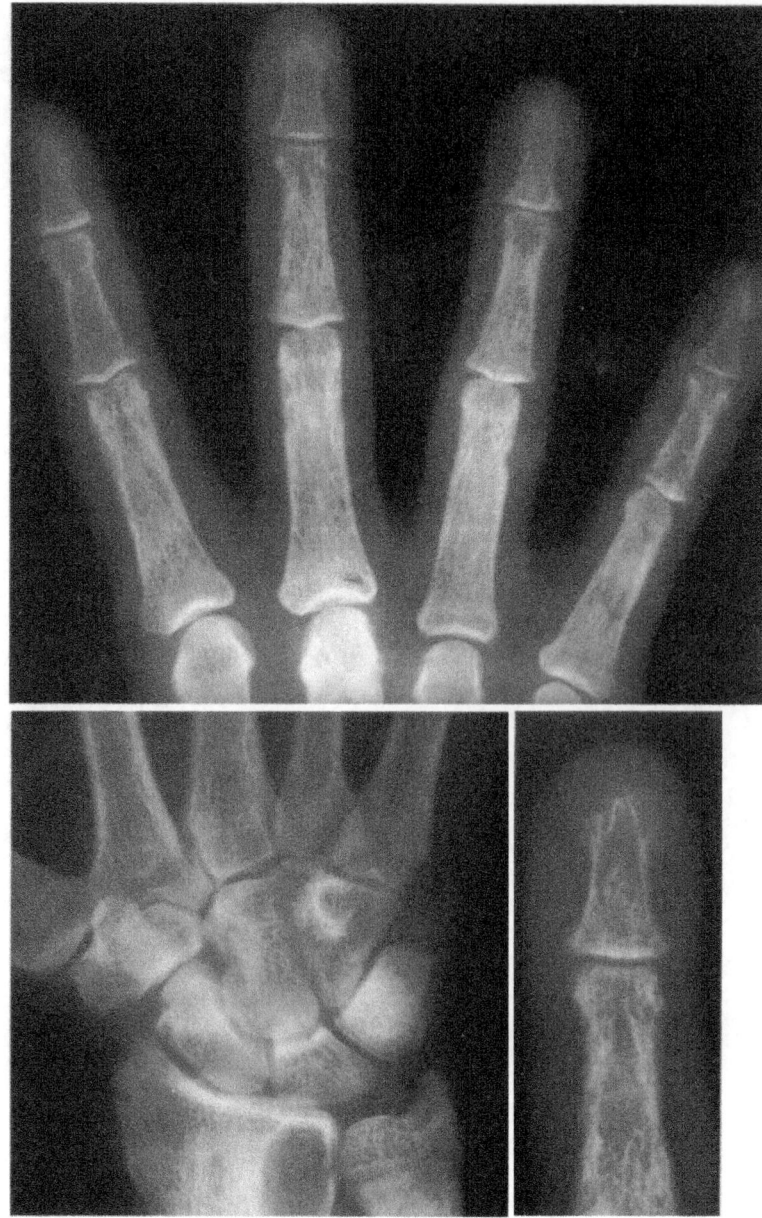

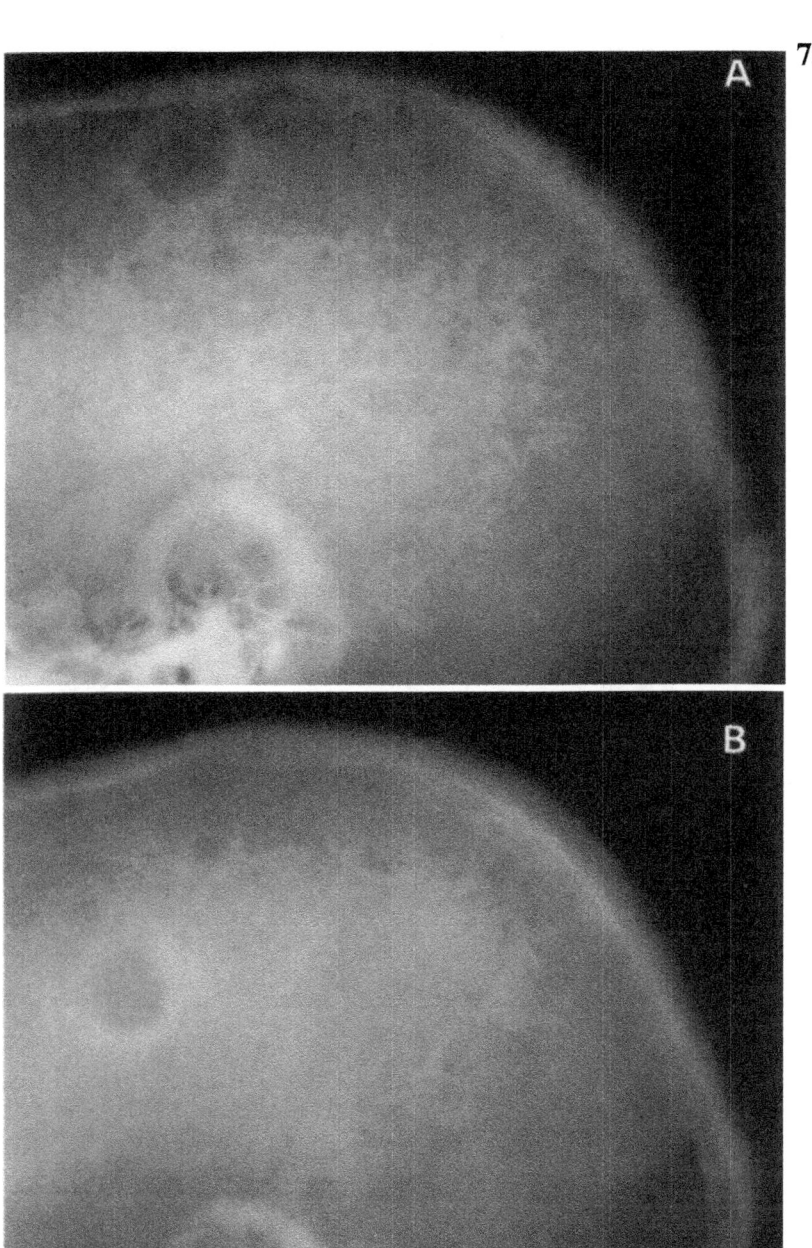

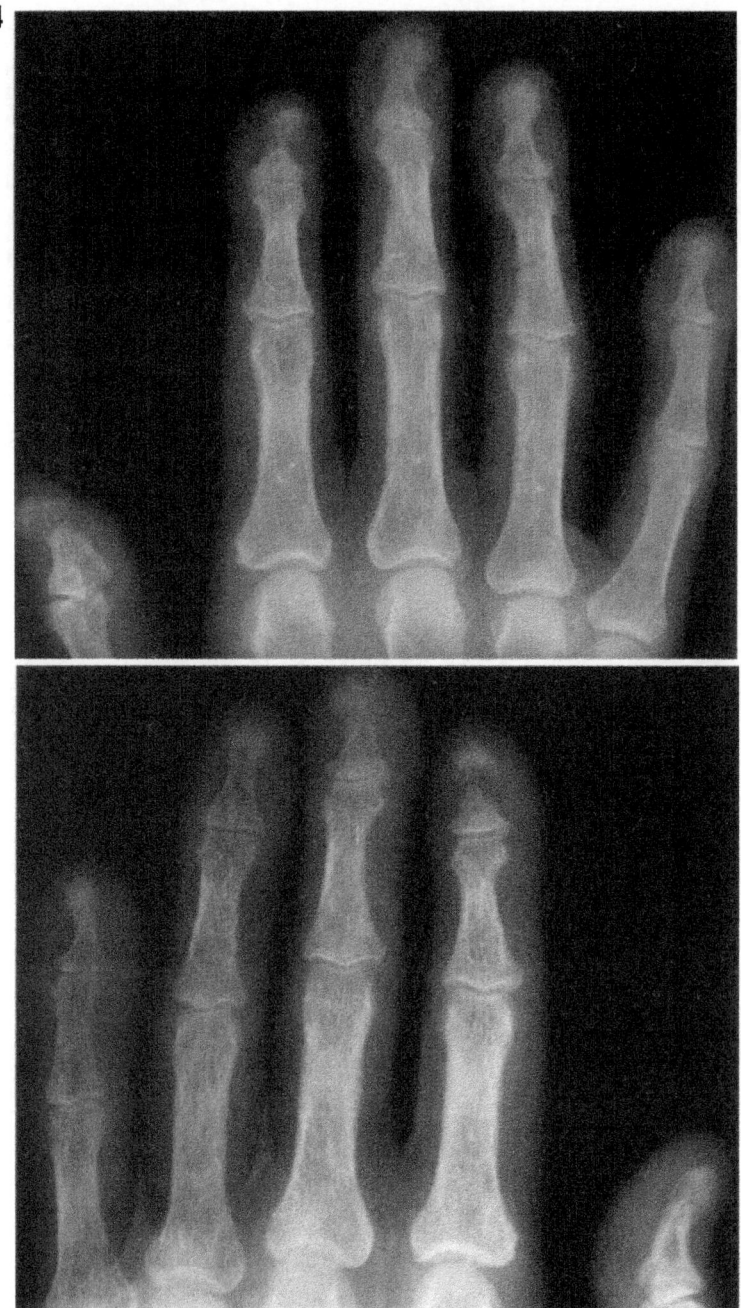

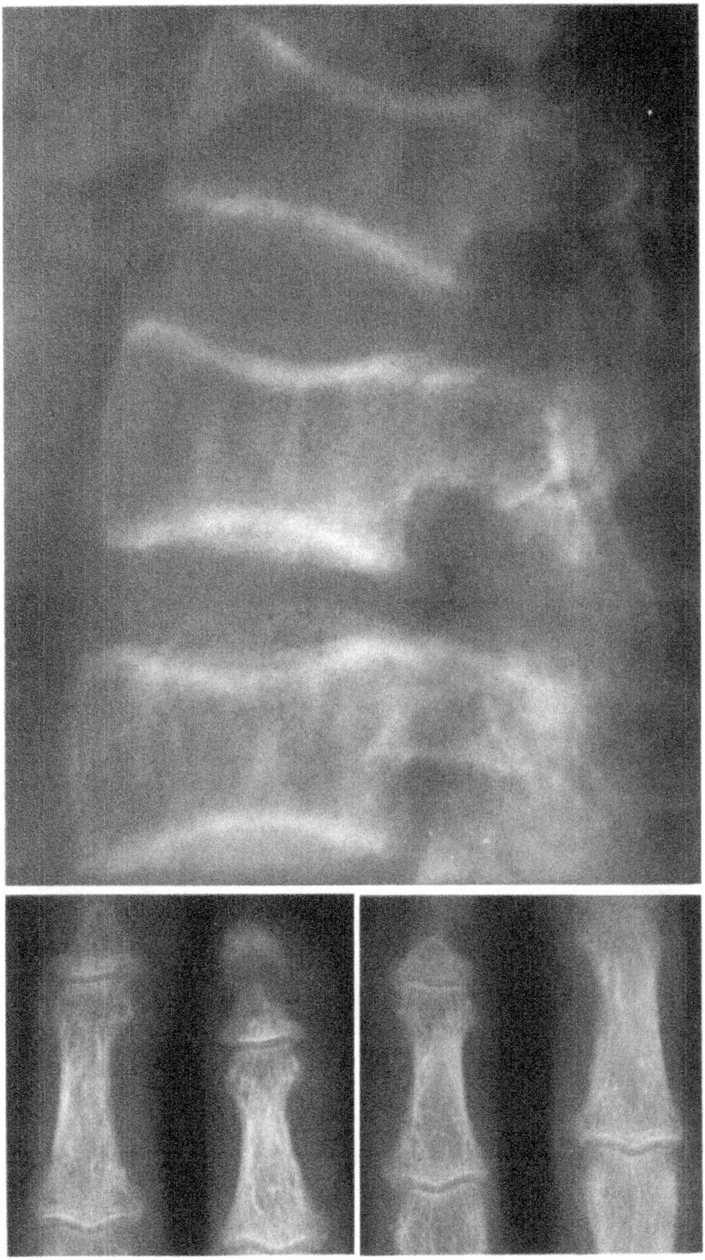

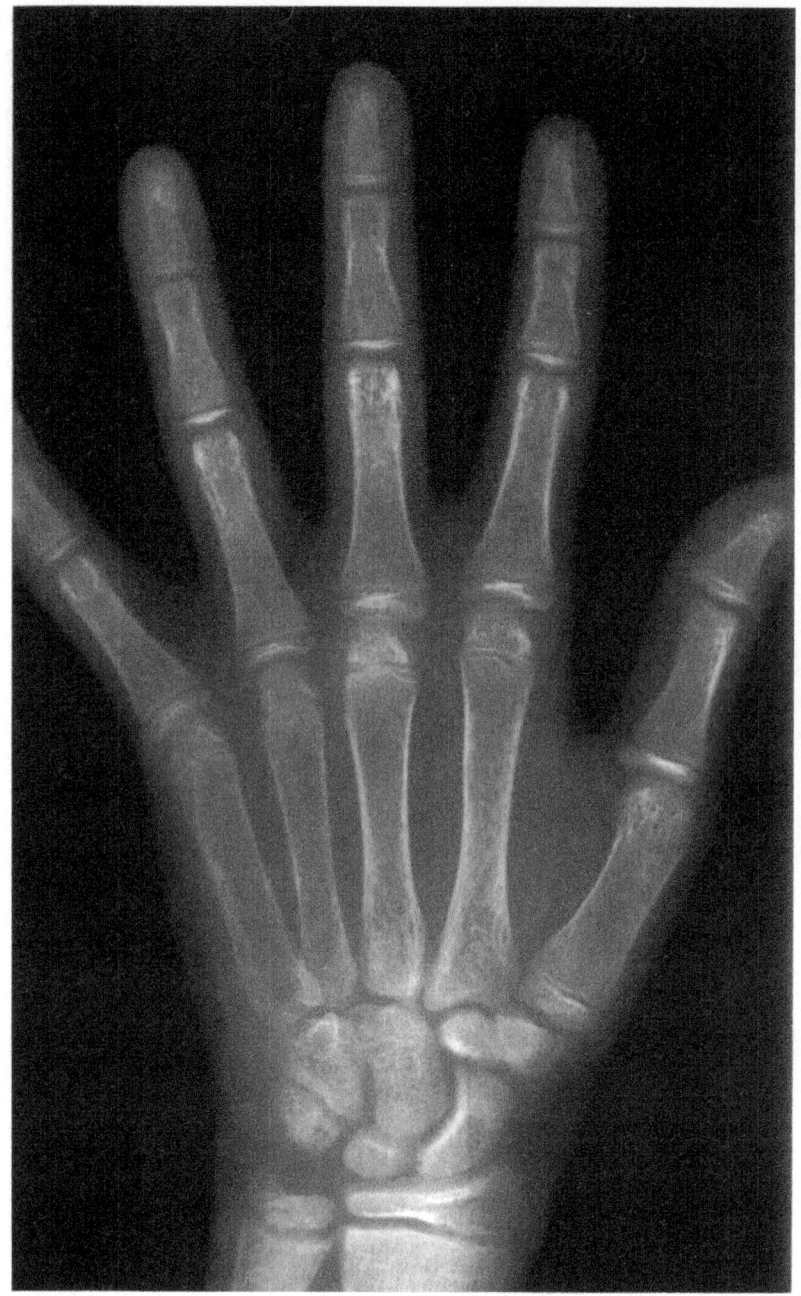

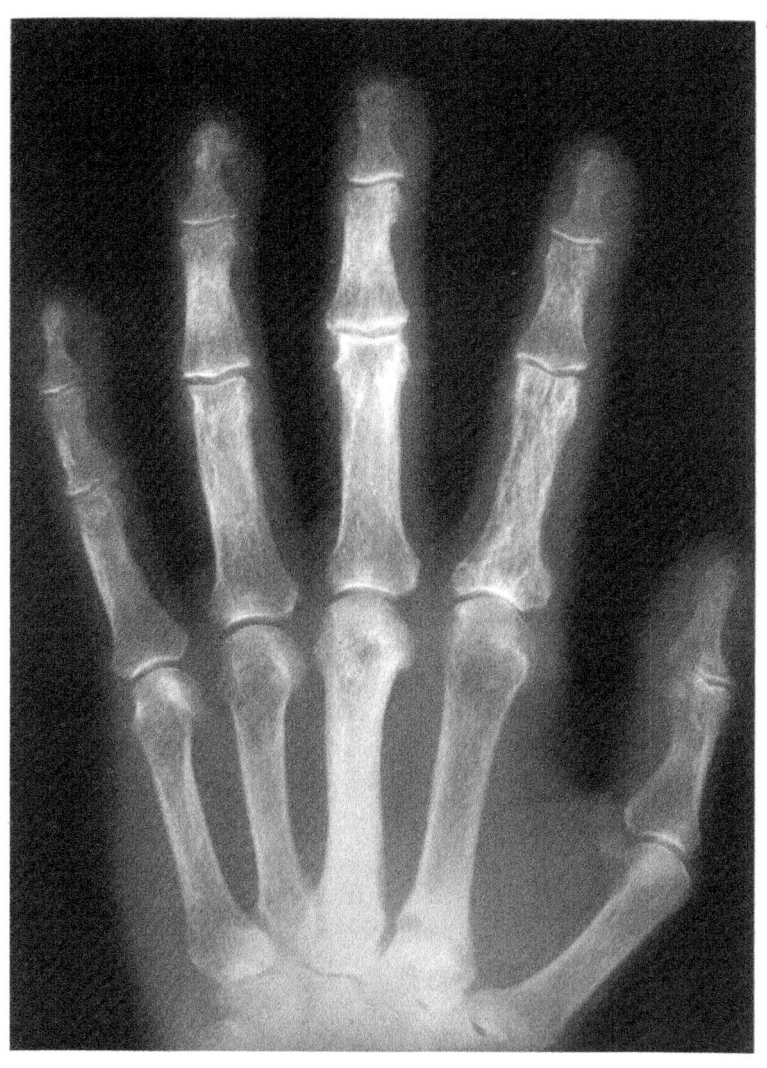

77

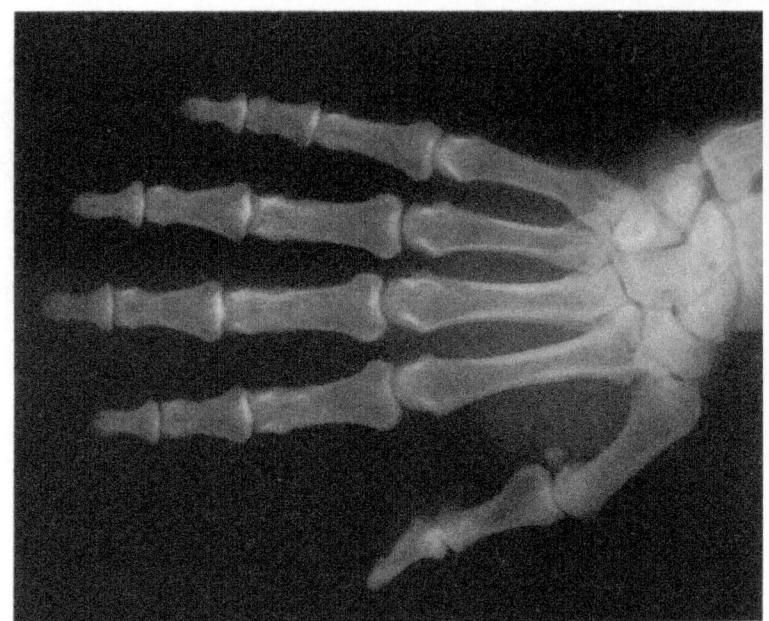
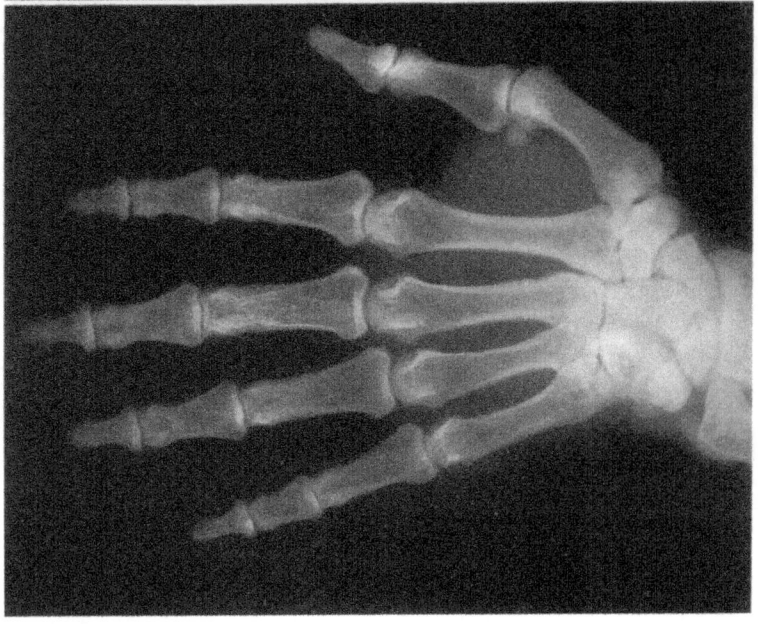

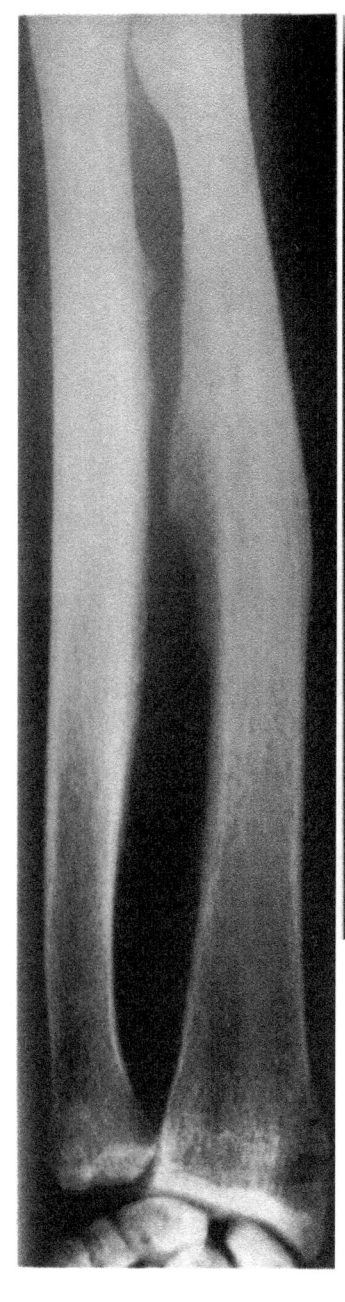
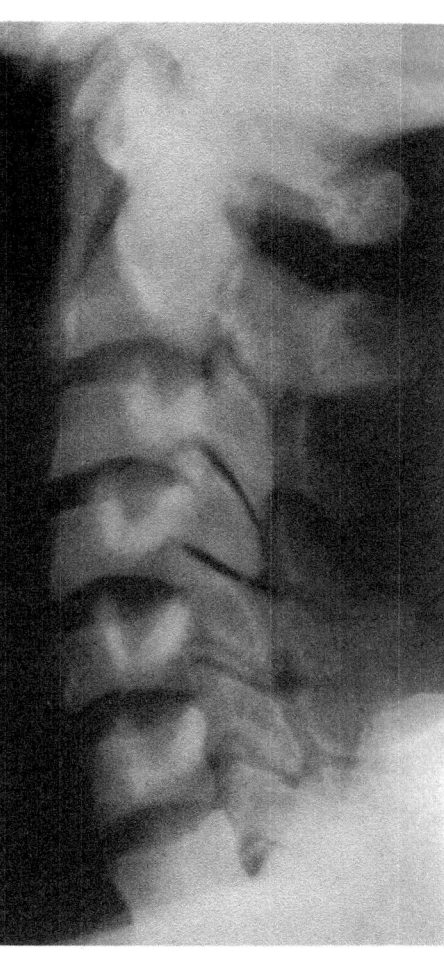

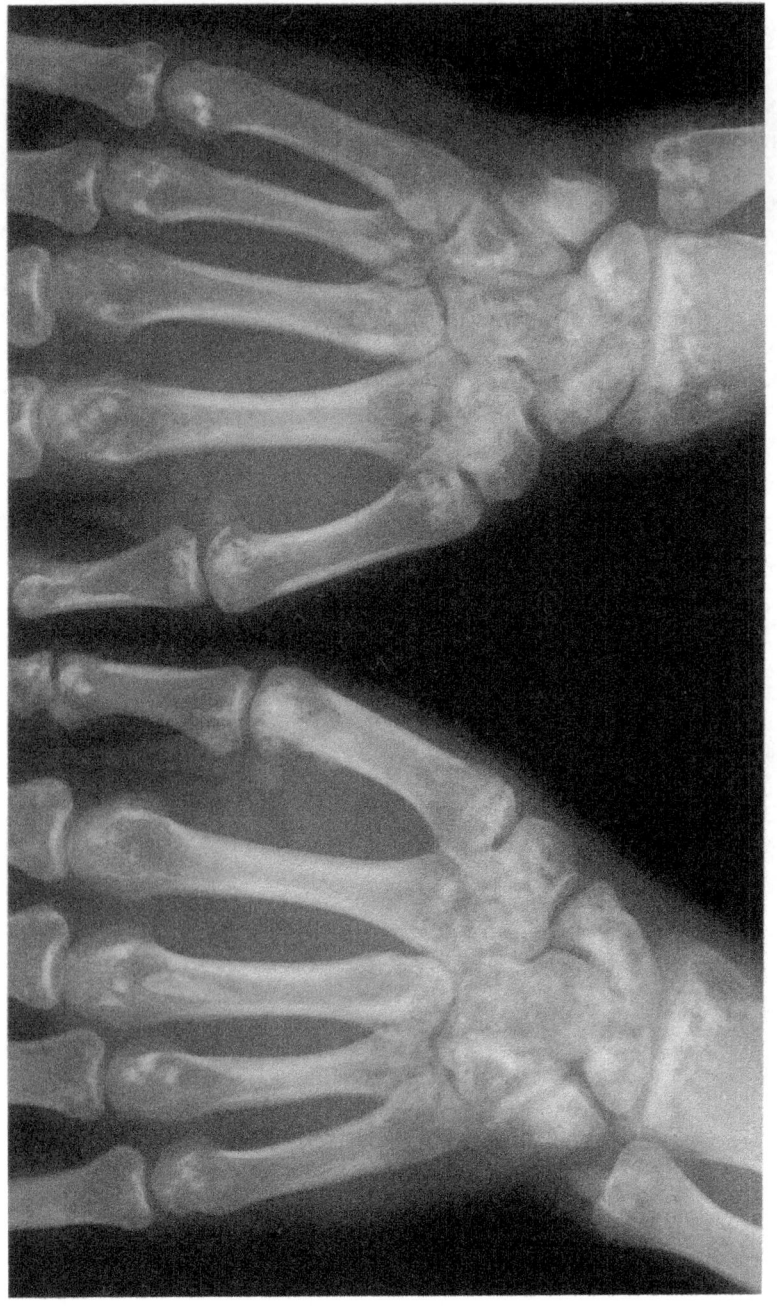

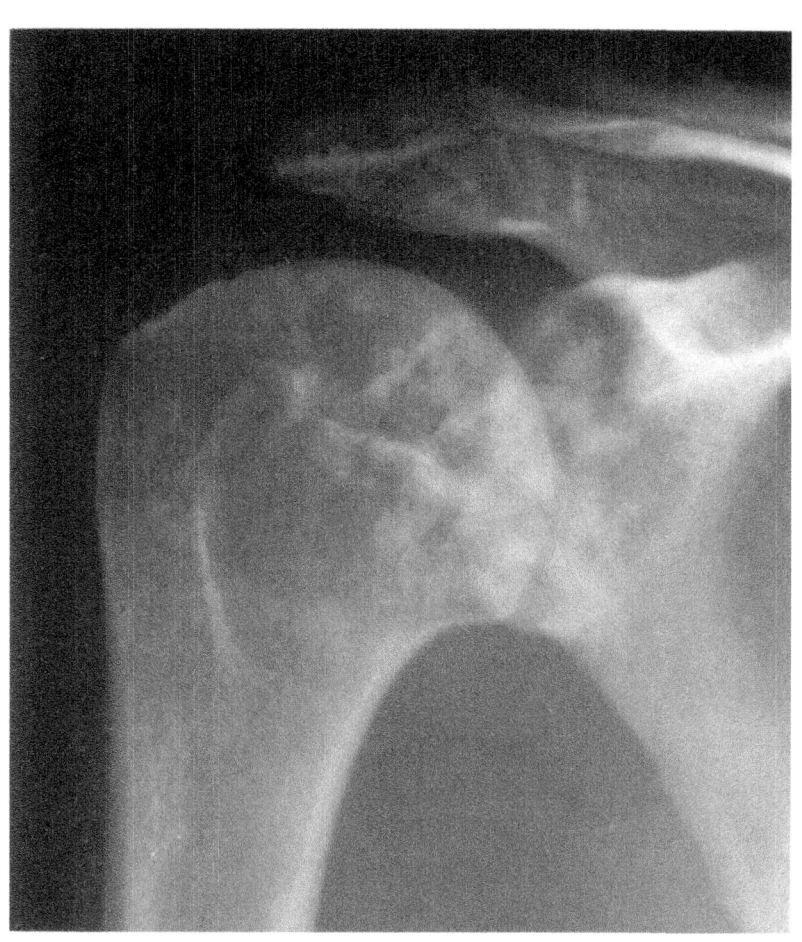

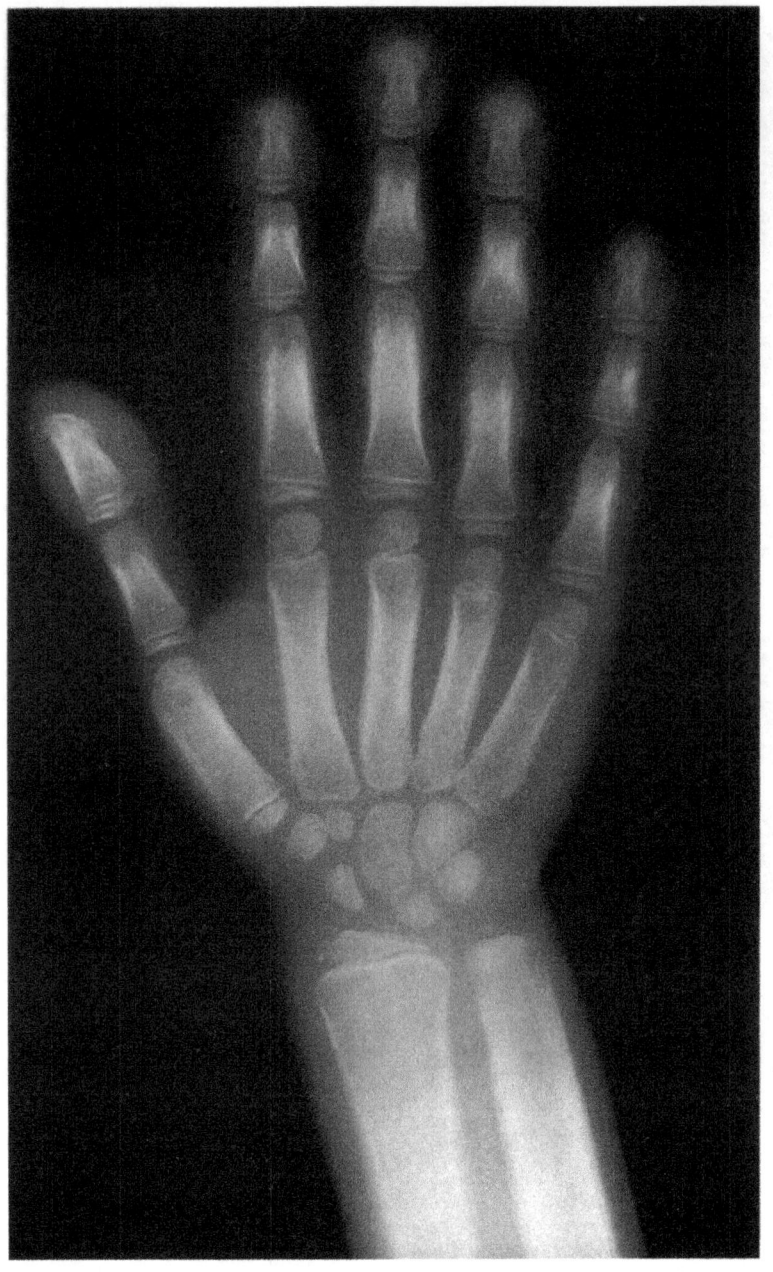

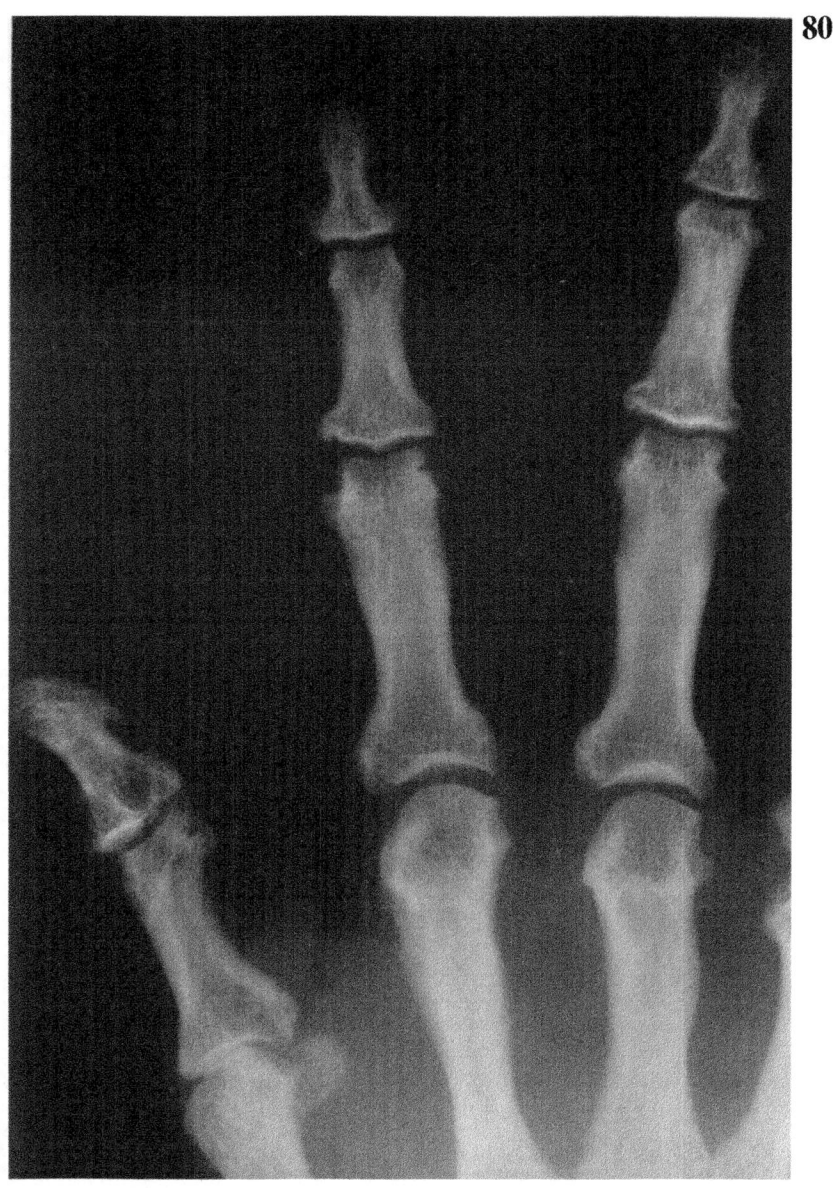

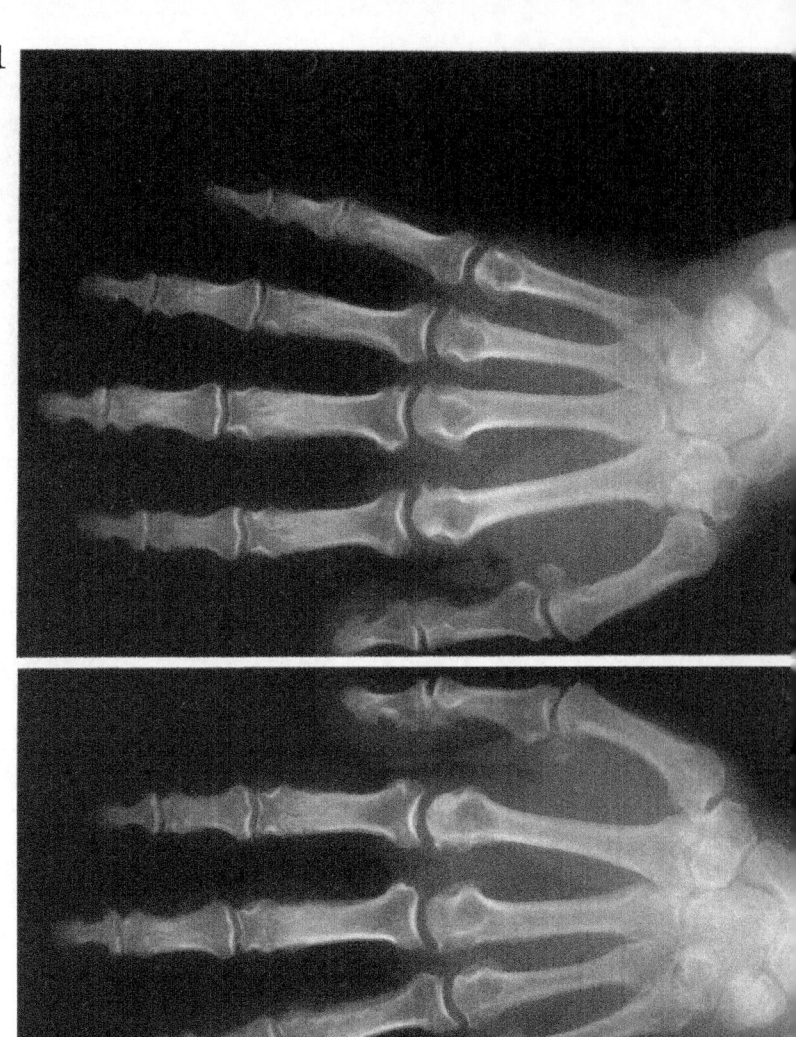

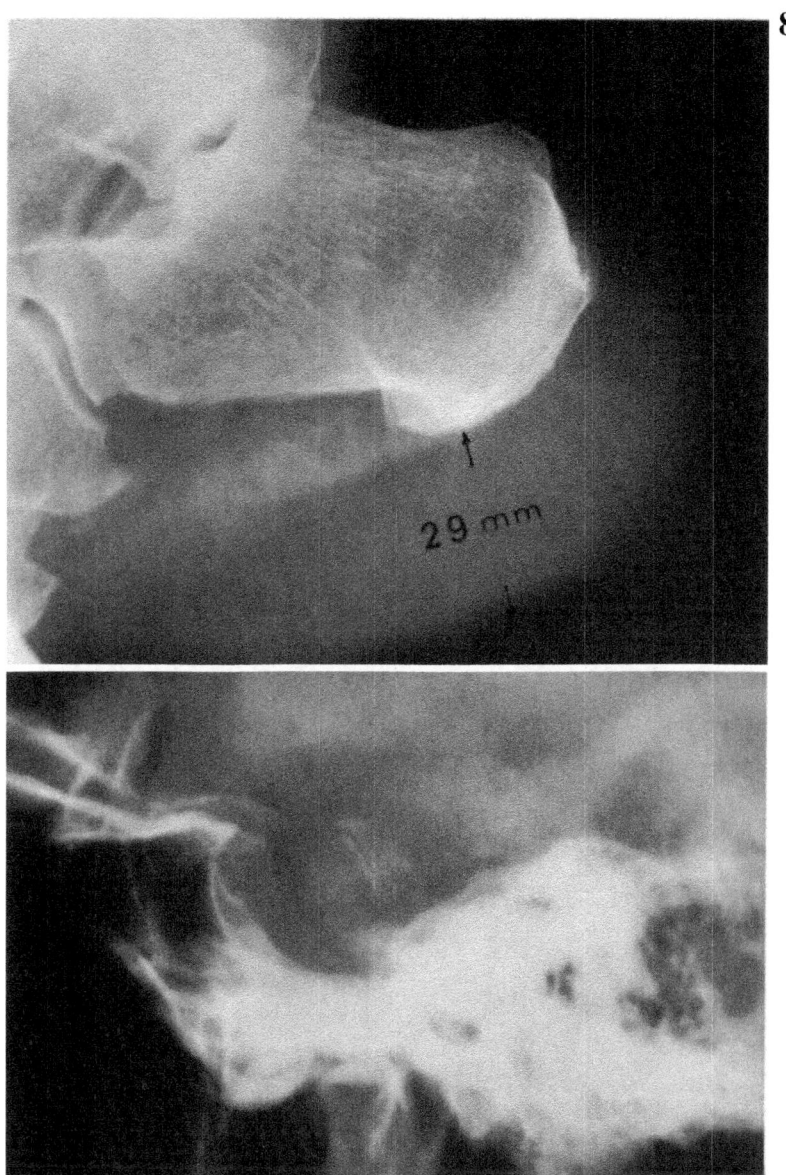

29 mm

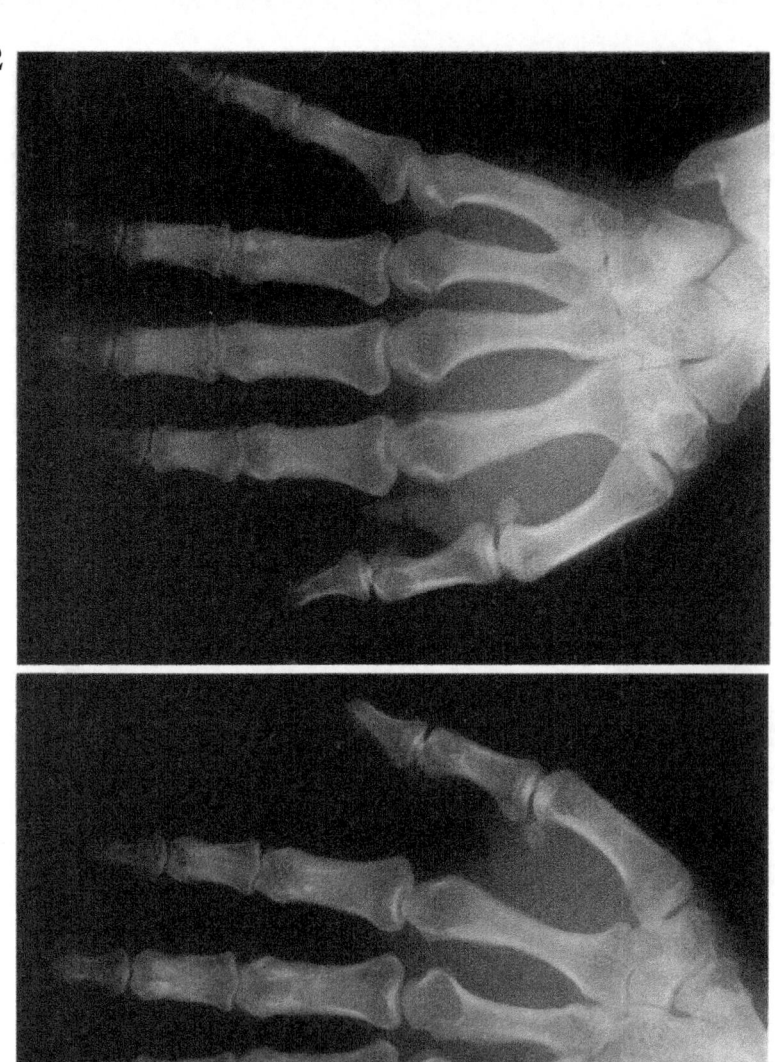

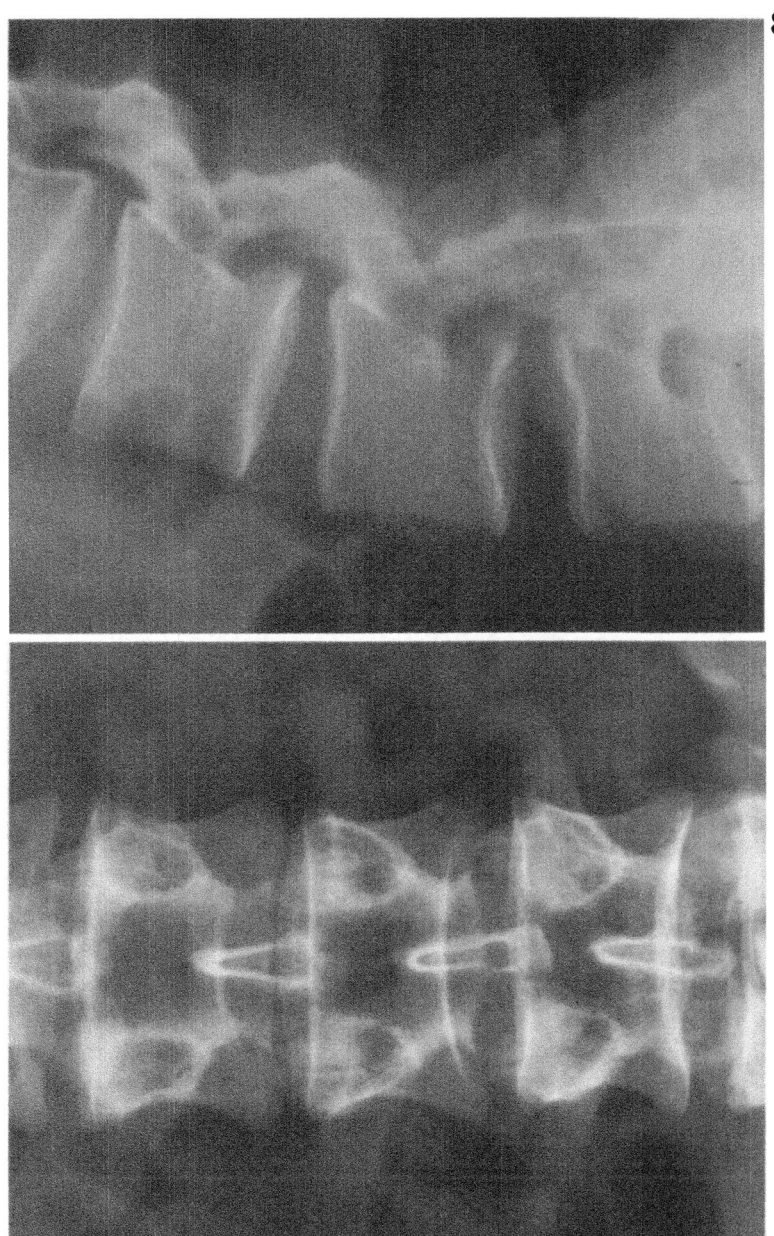

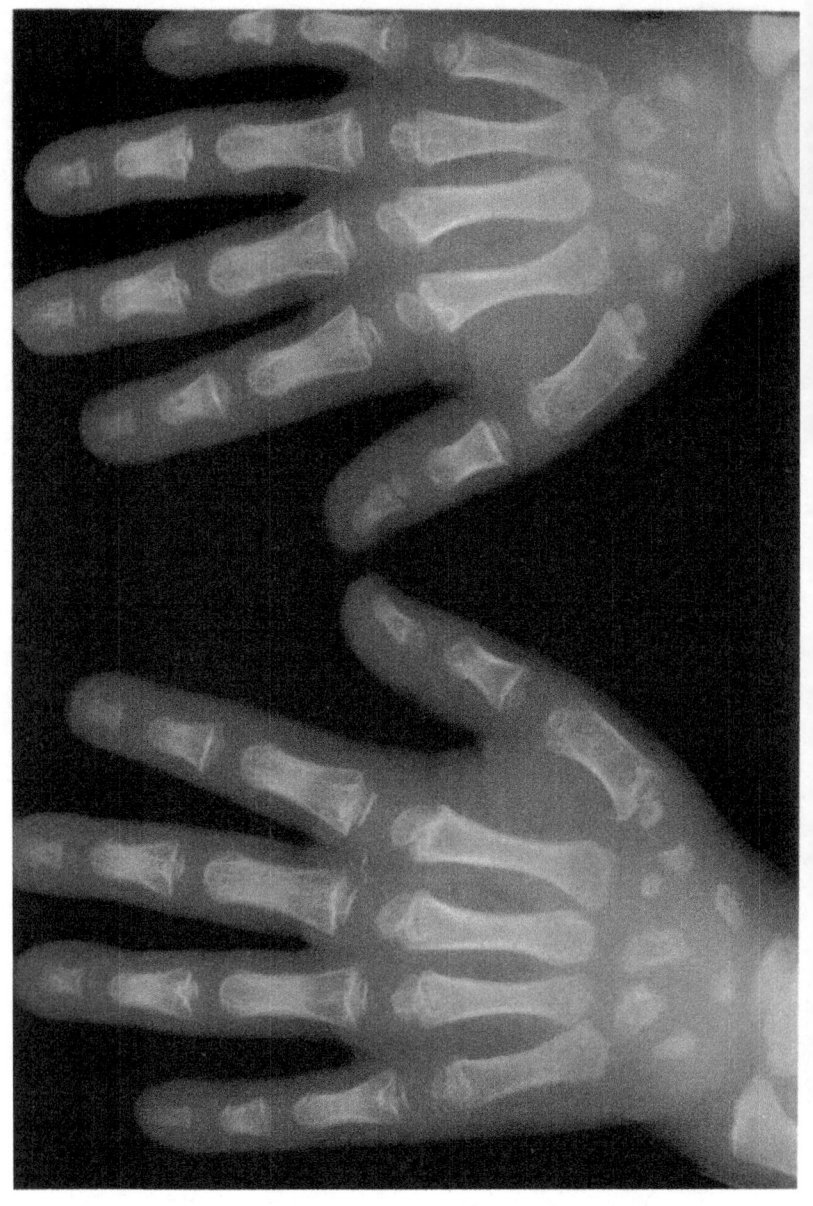

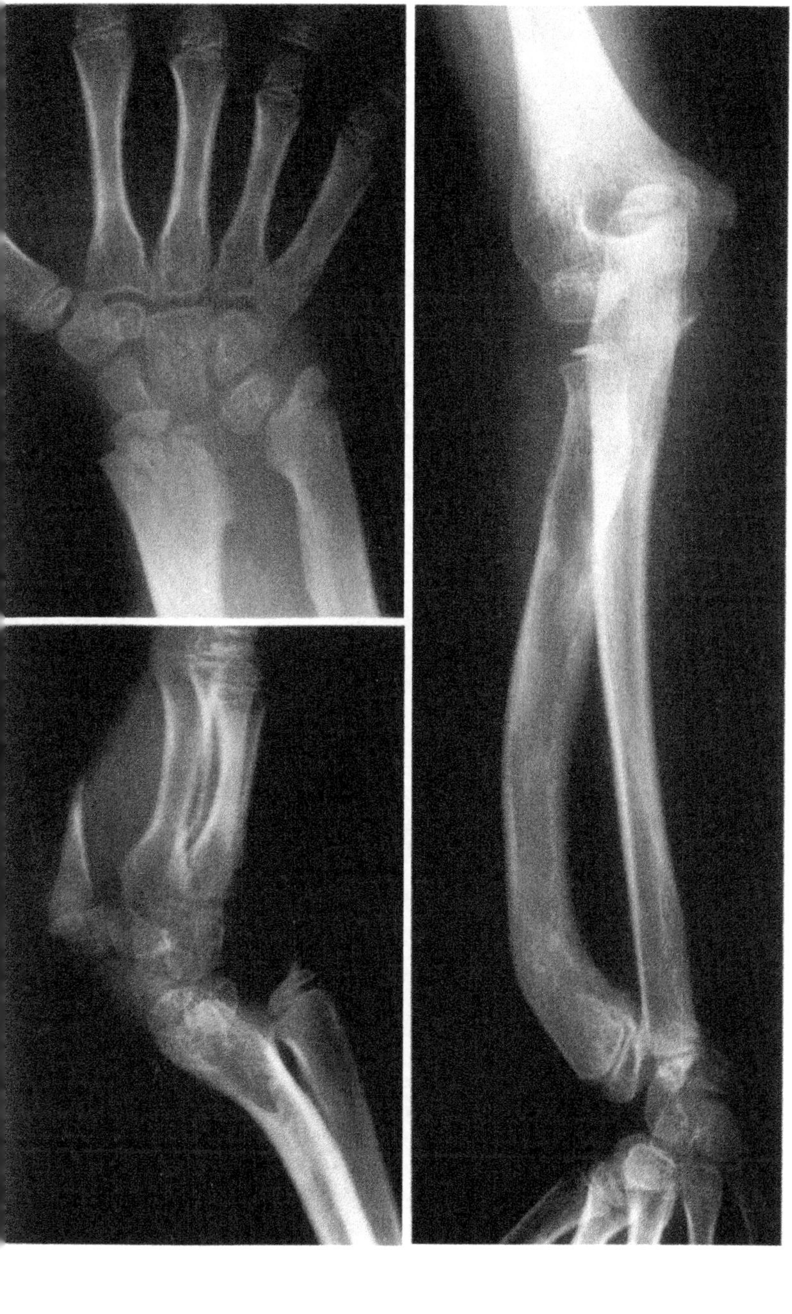

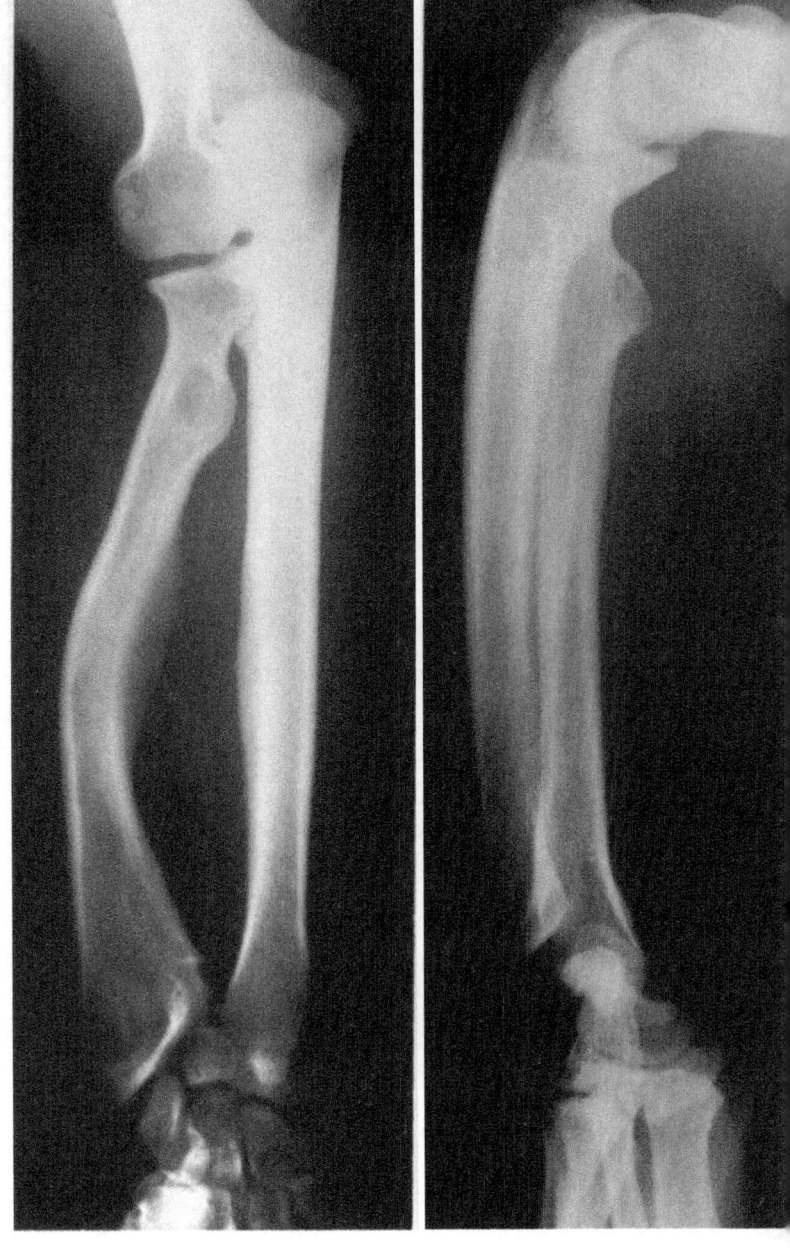

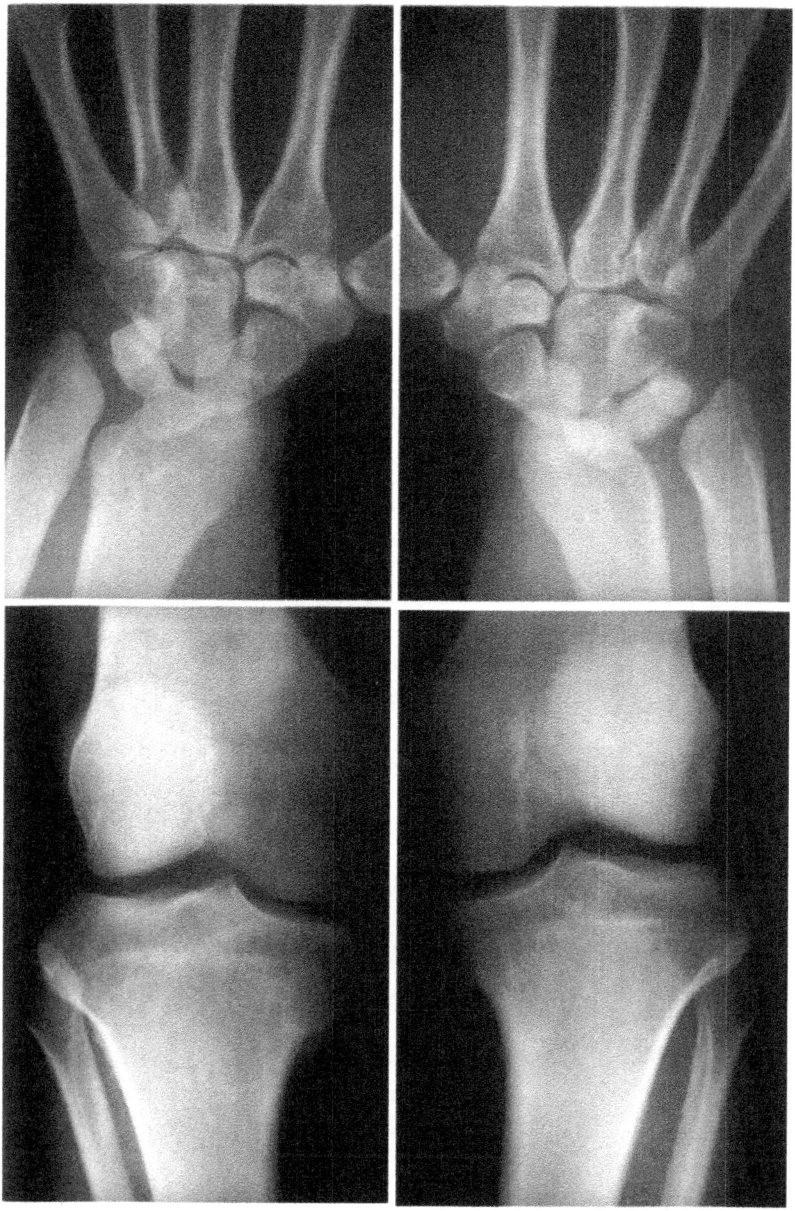

86

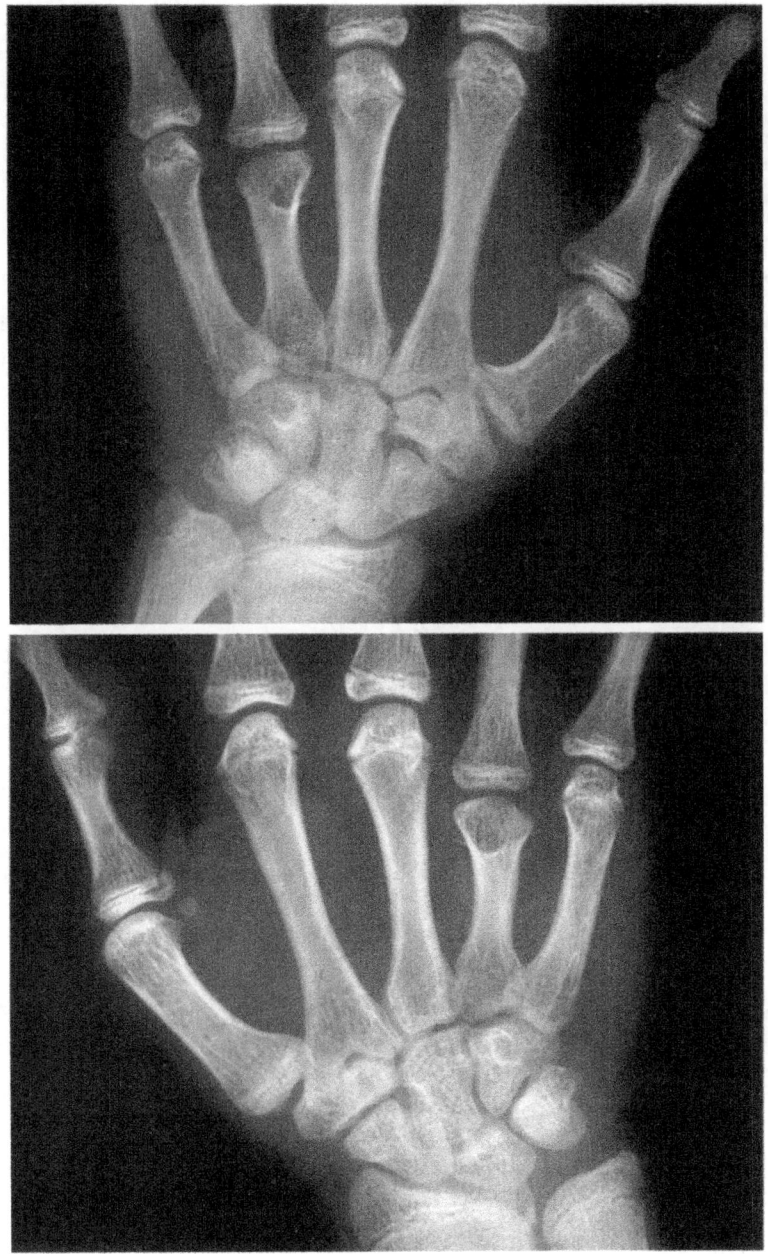

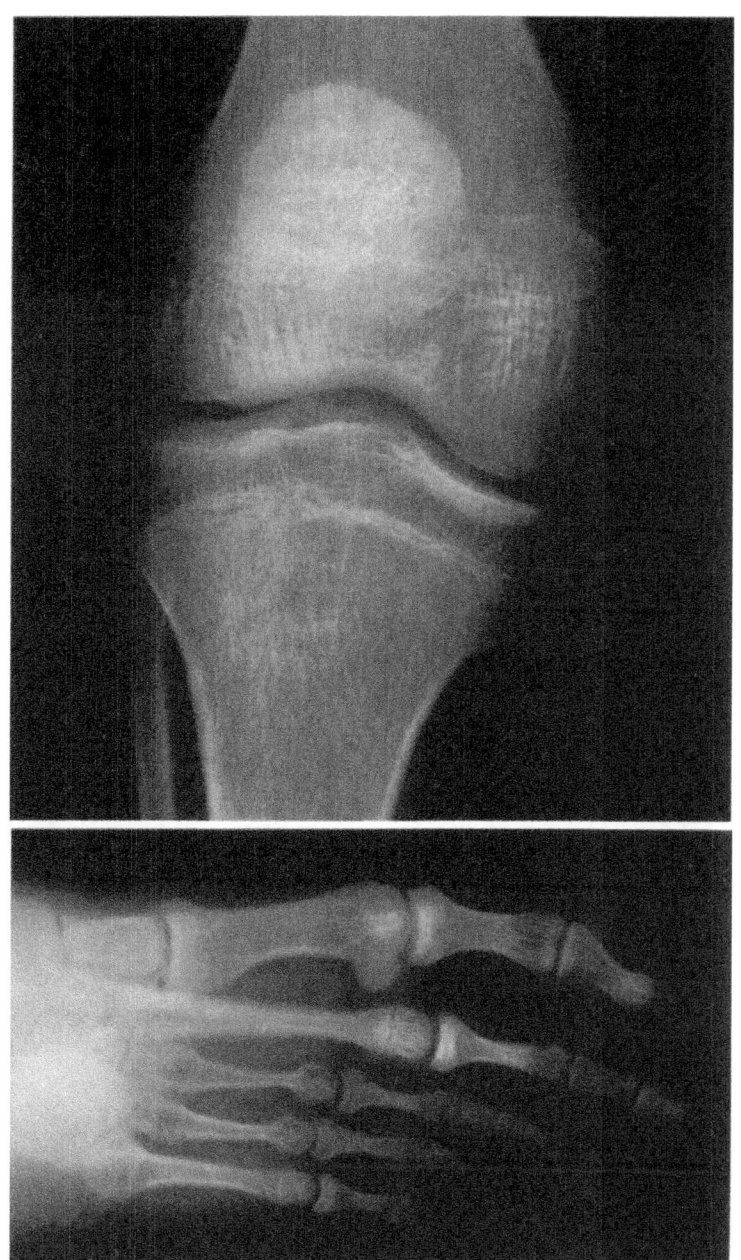

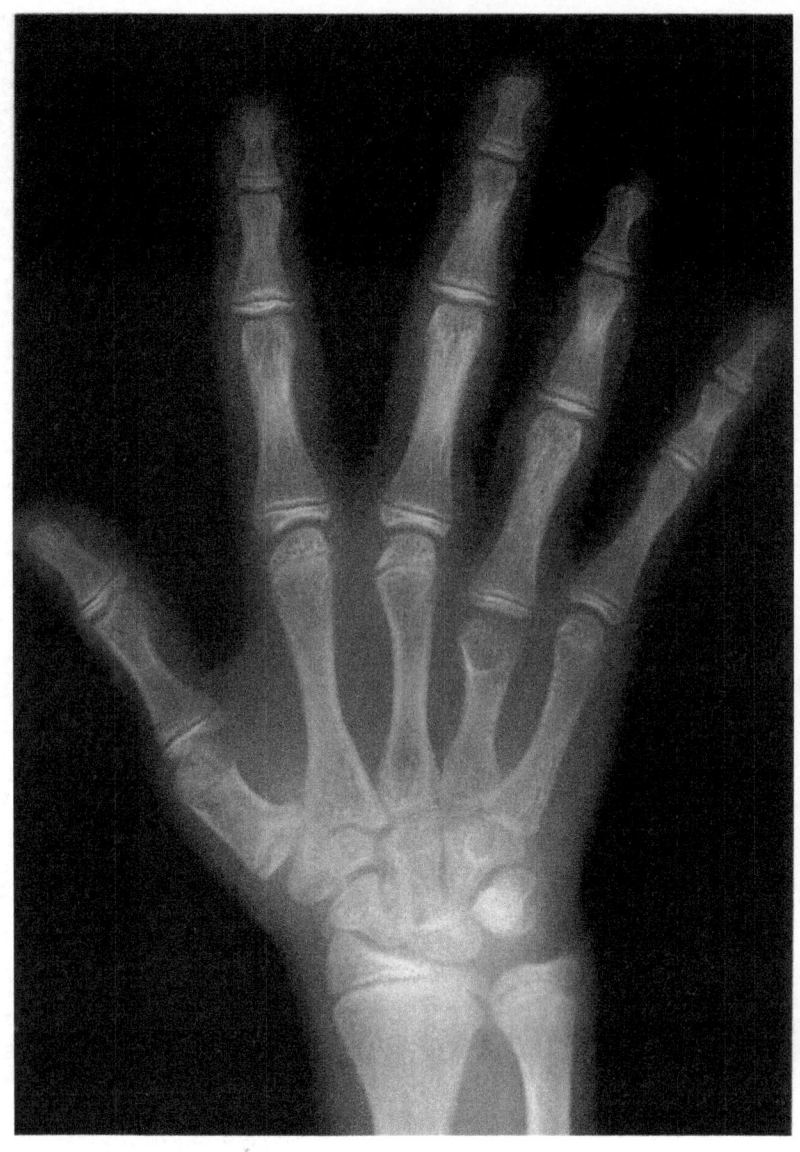

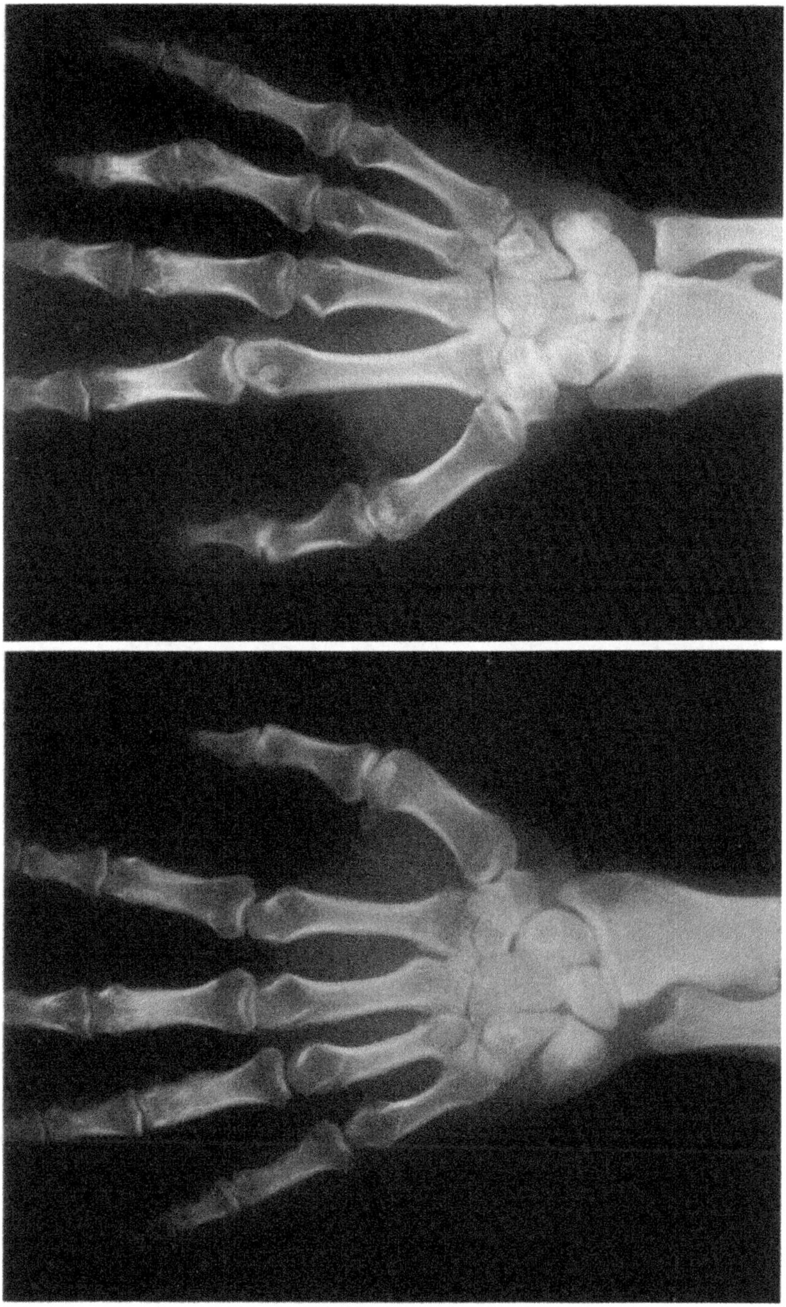

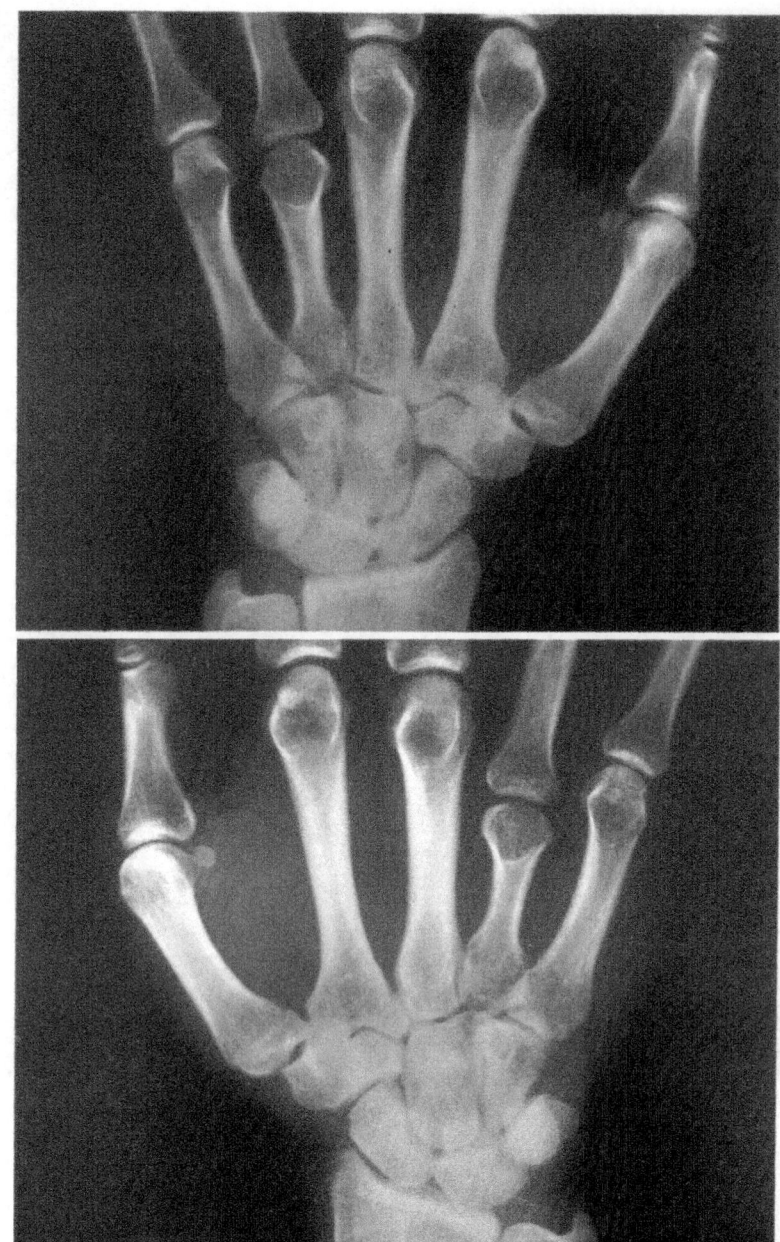

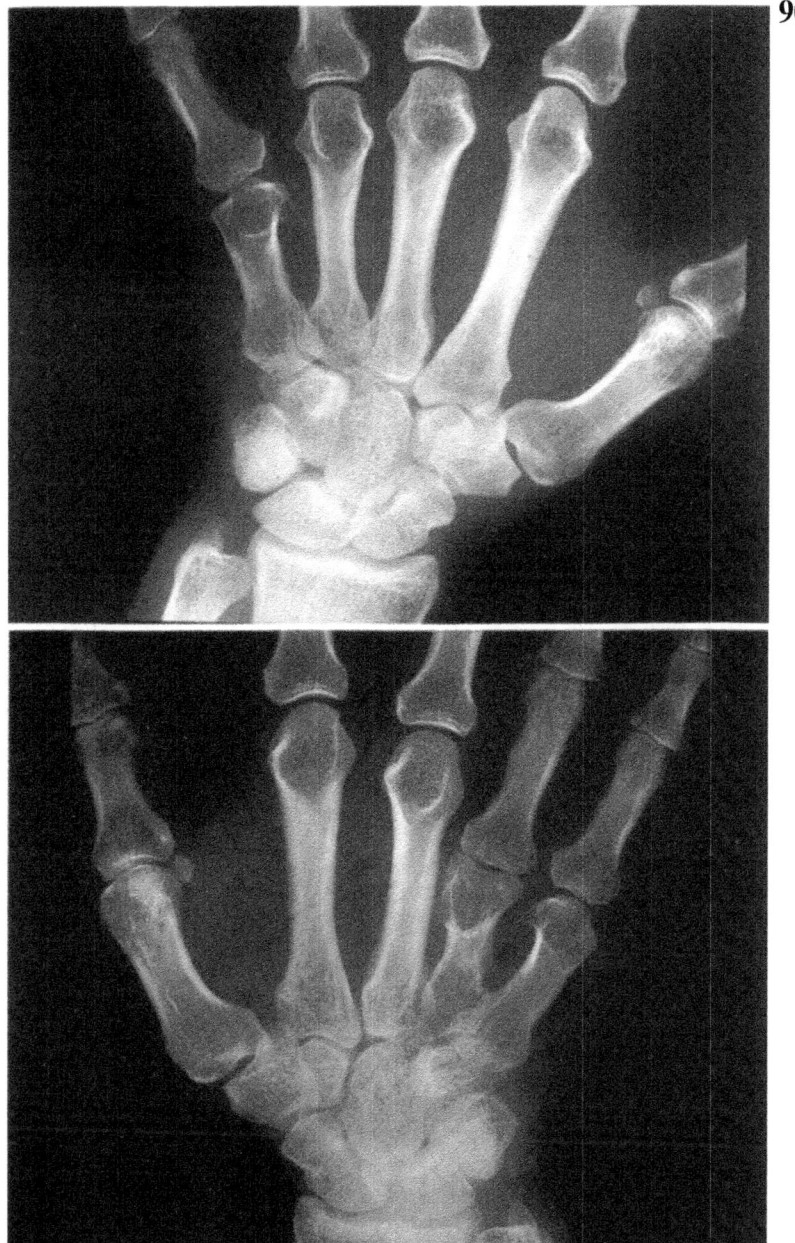

91

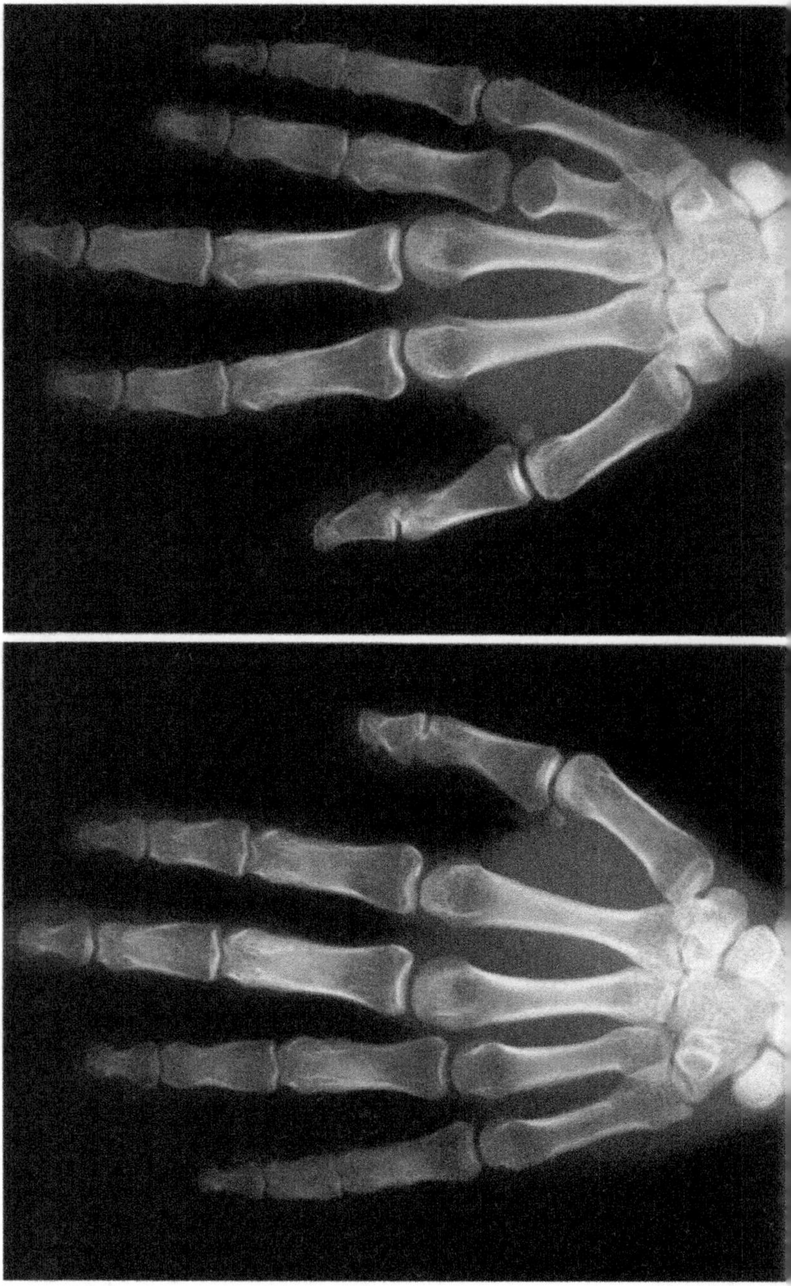

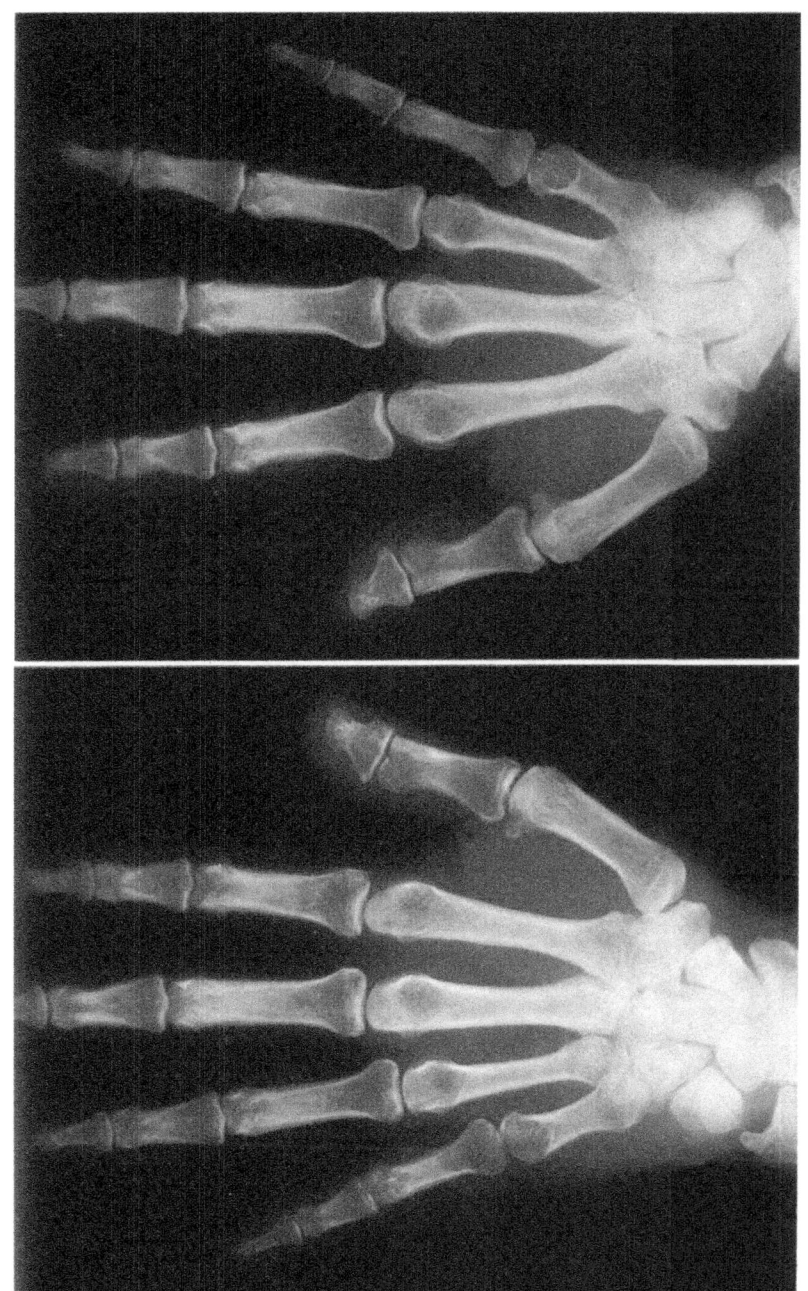

93

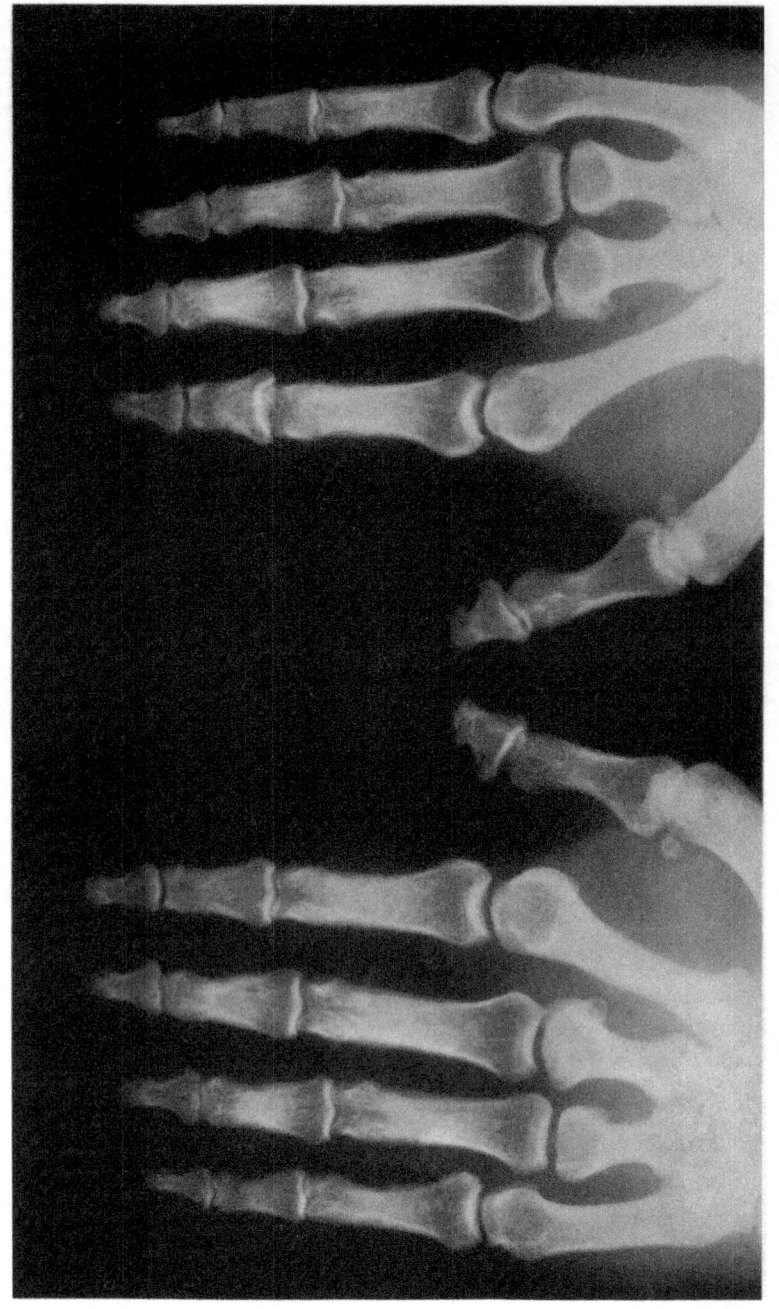

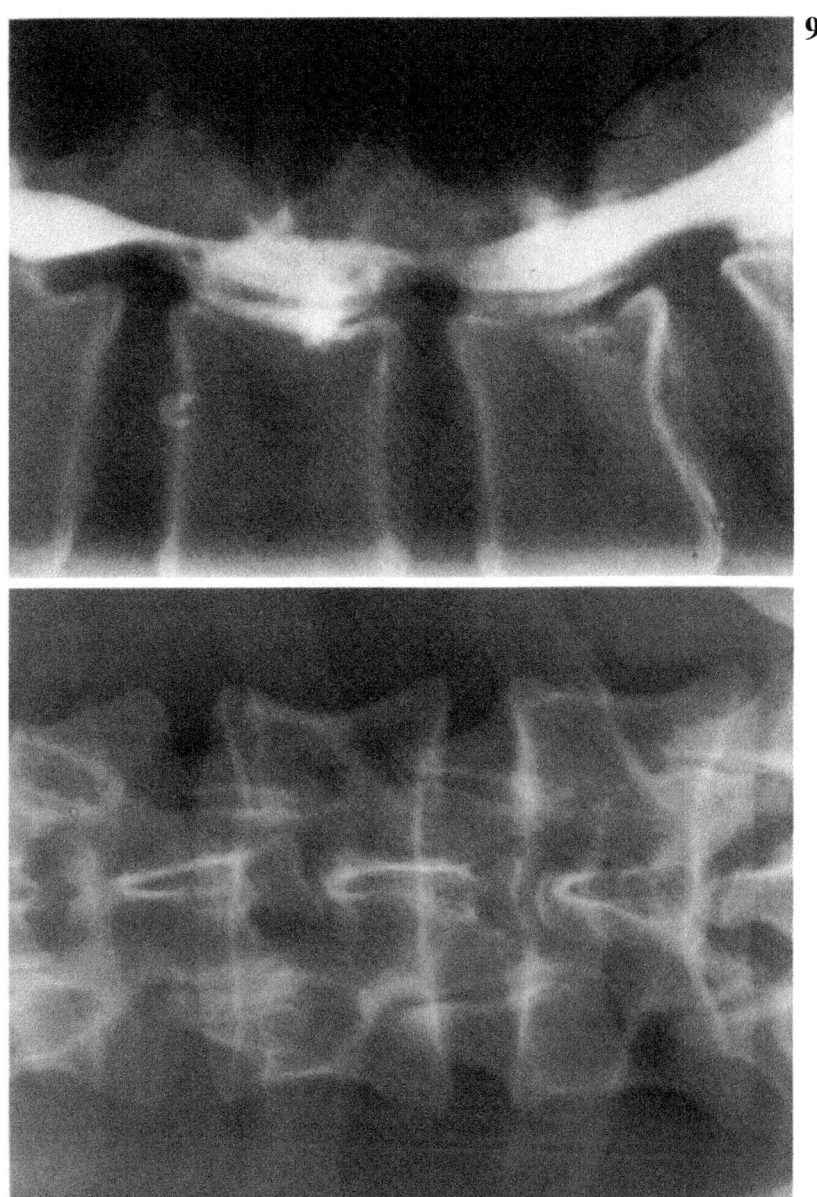

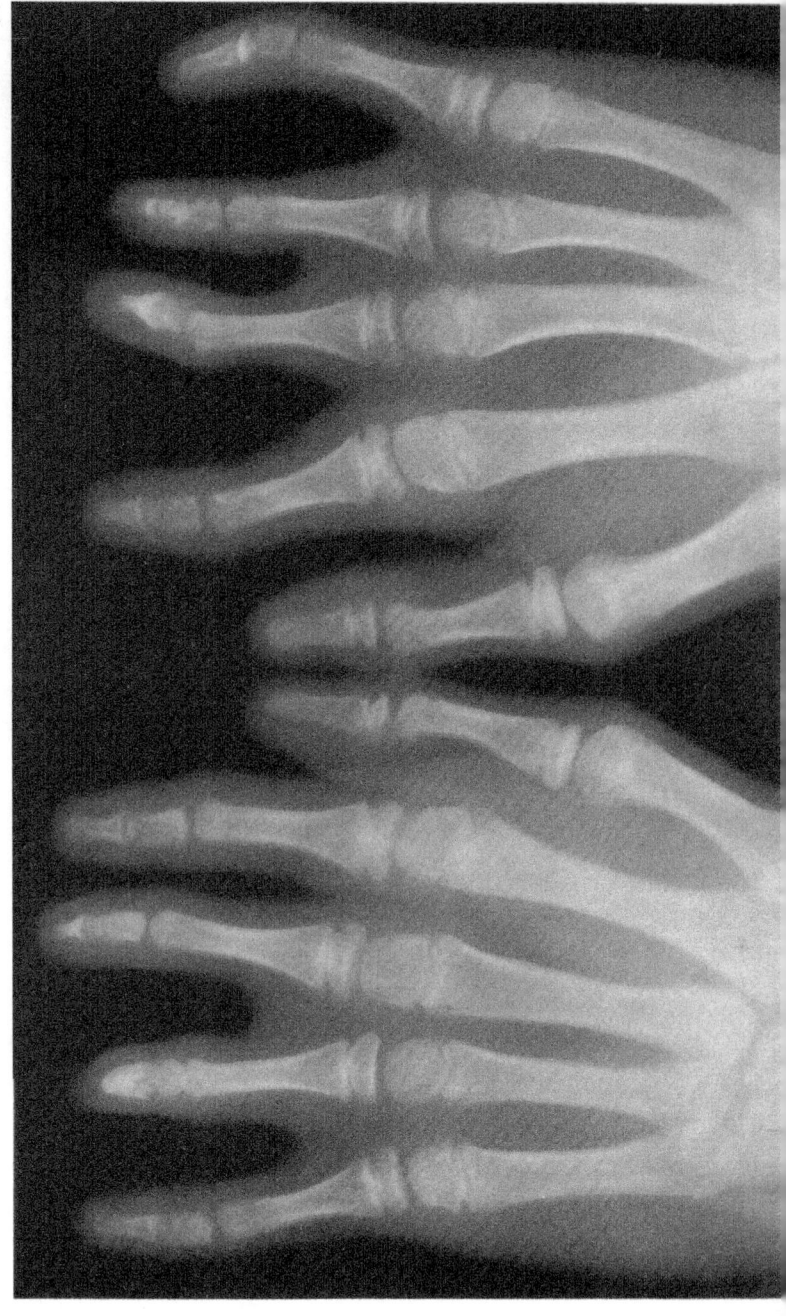

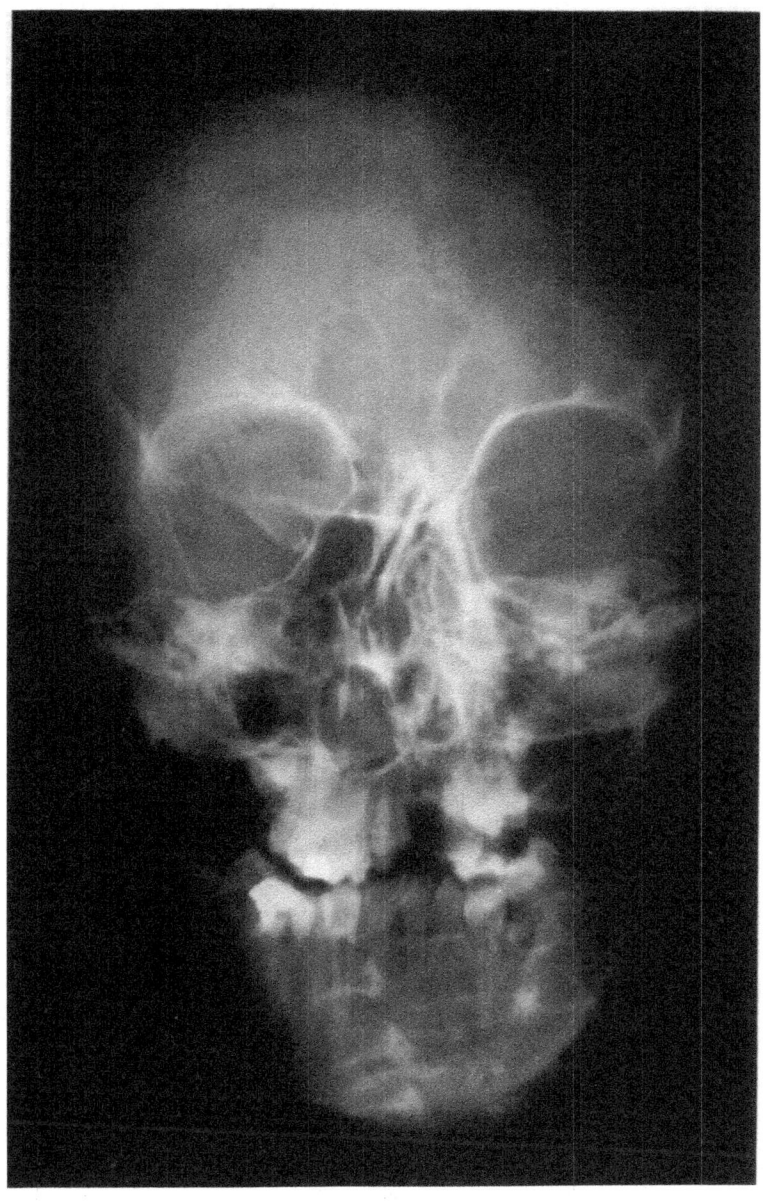

95

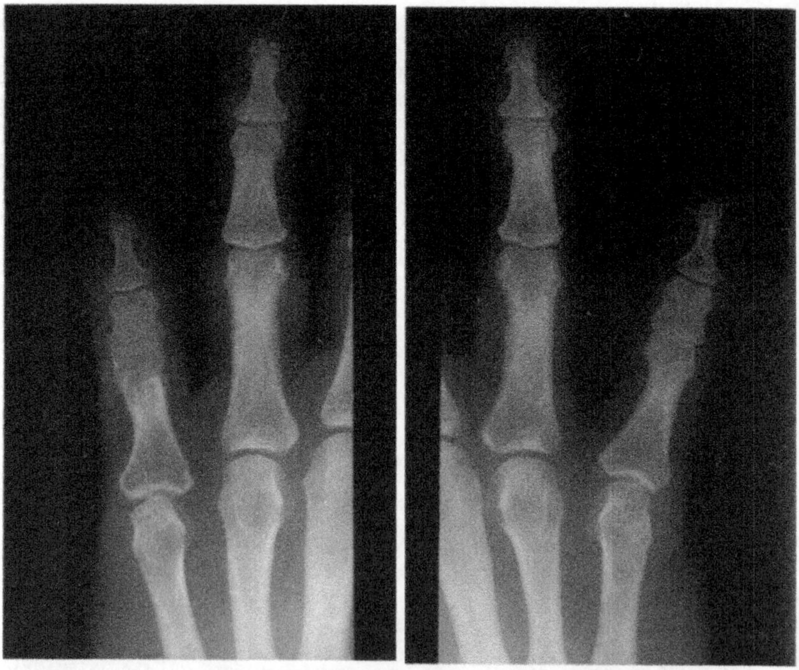

96

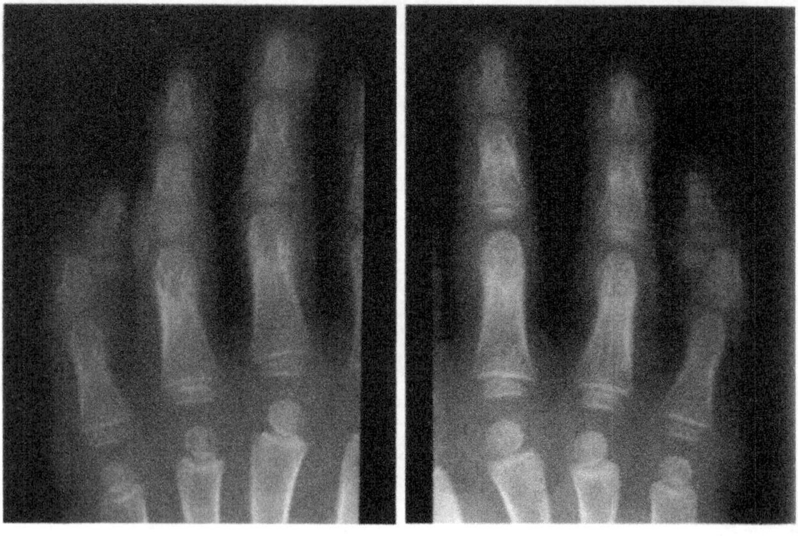

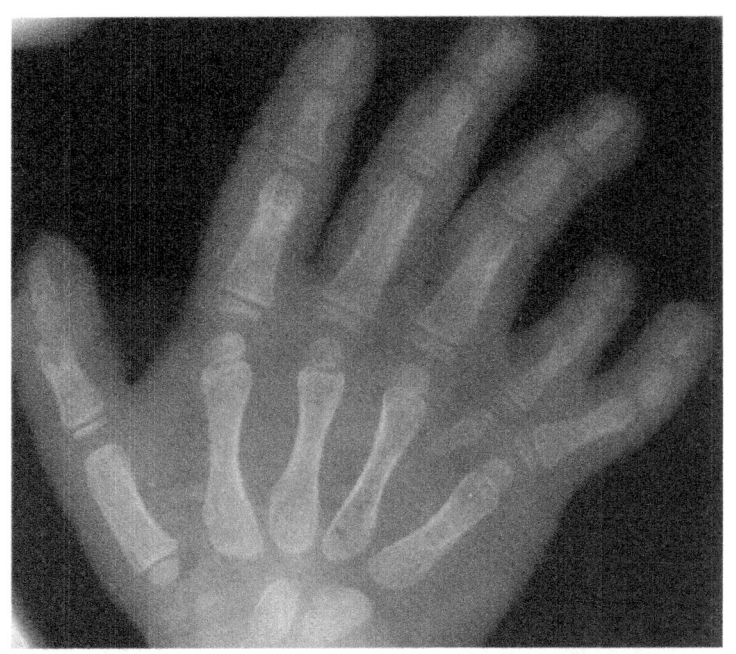

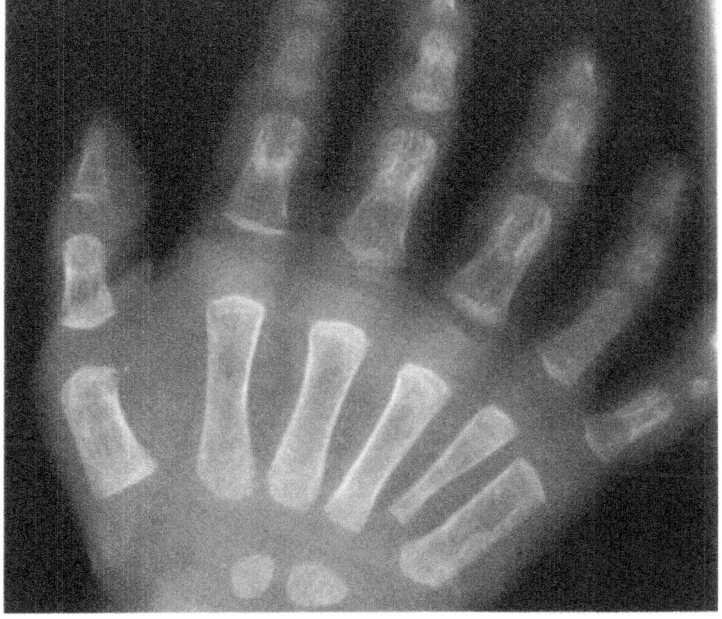

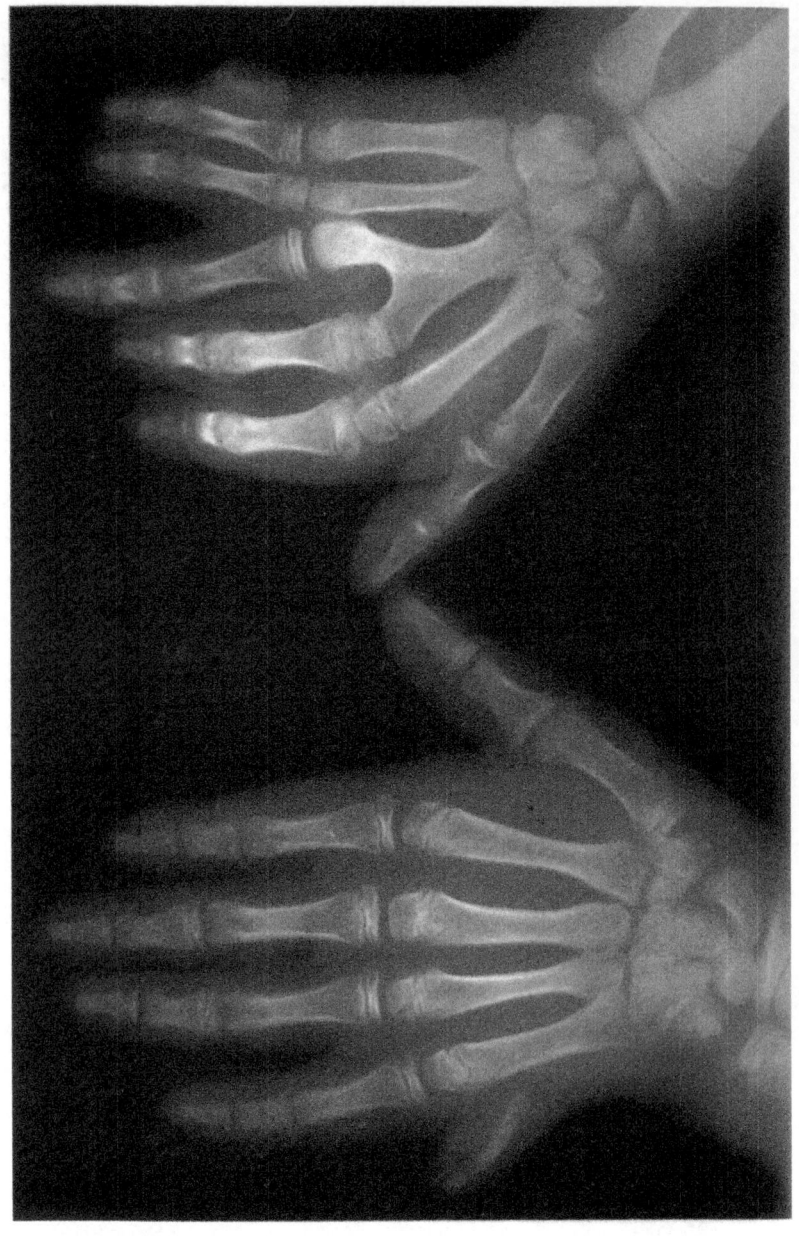

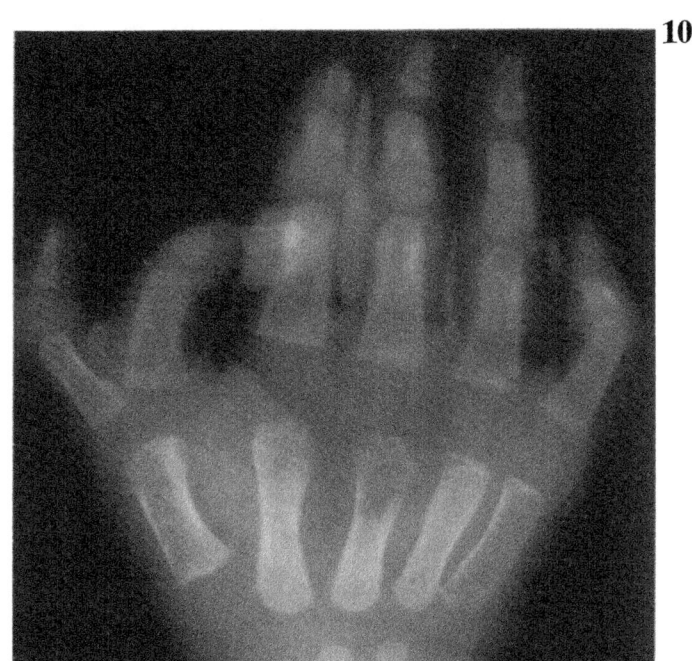

100

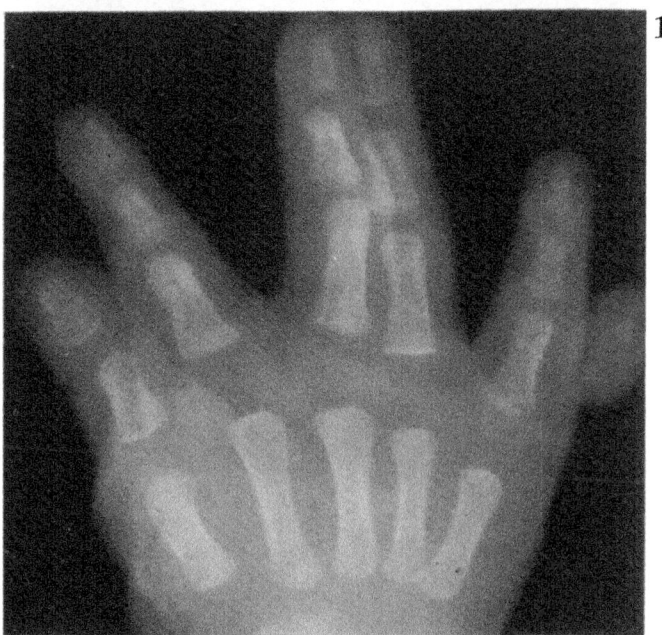

101

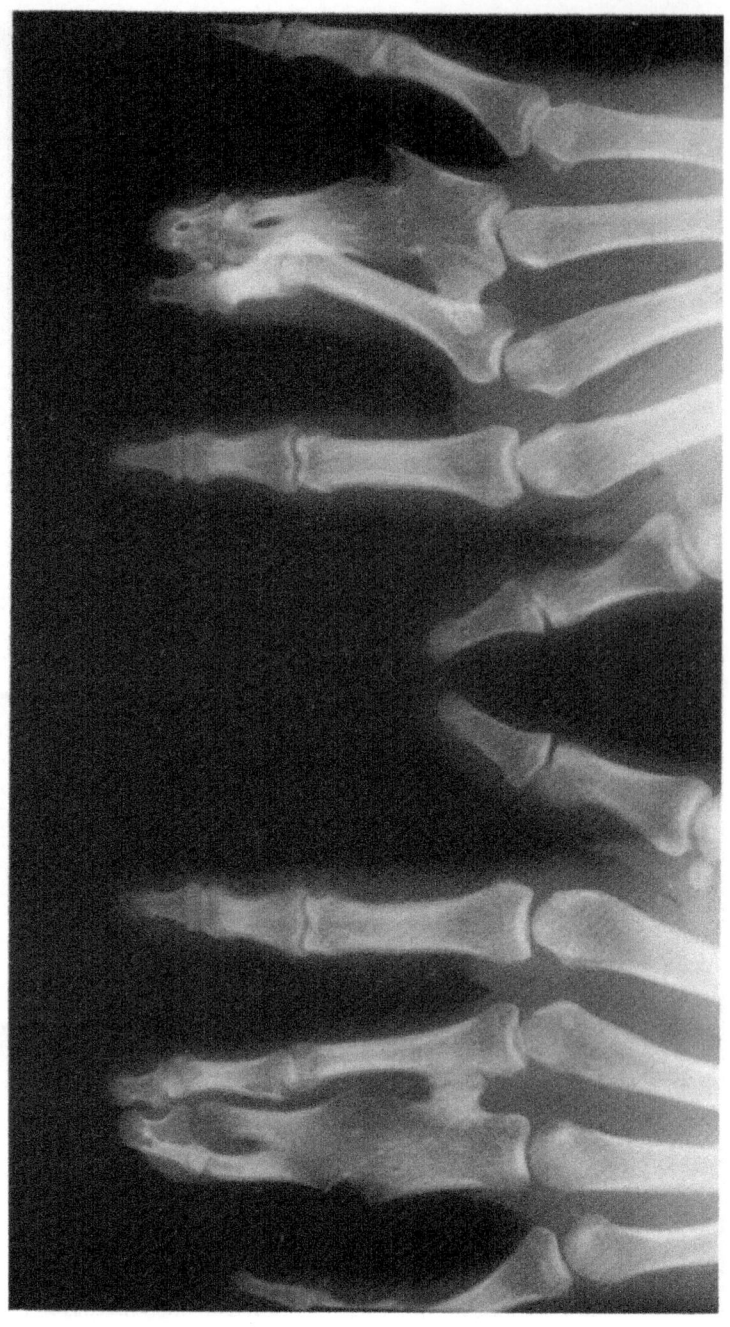

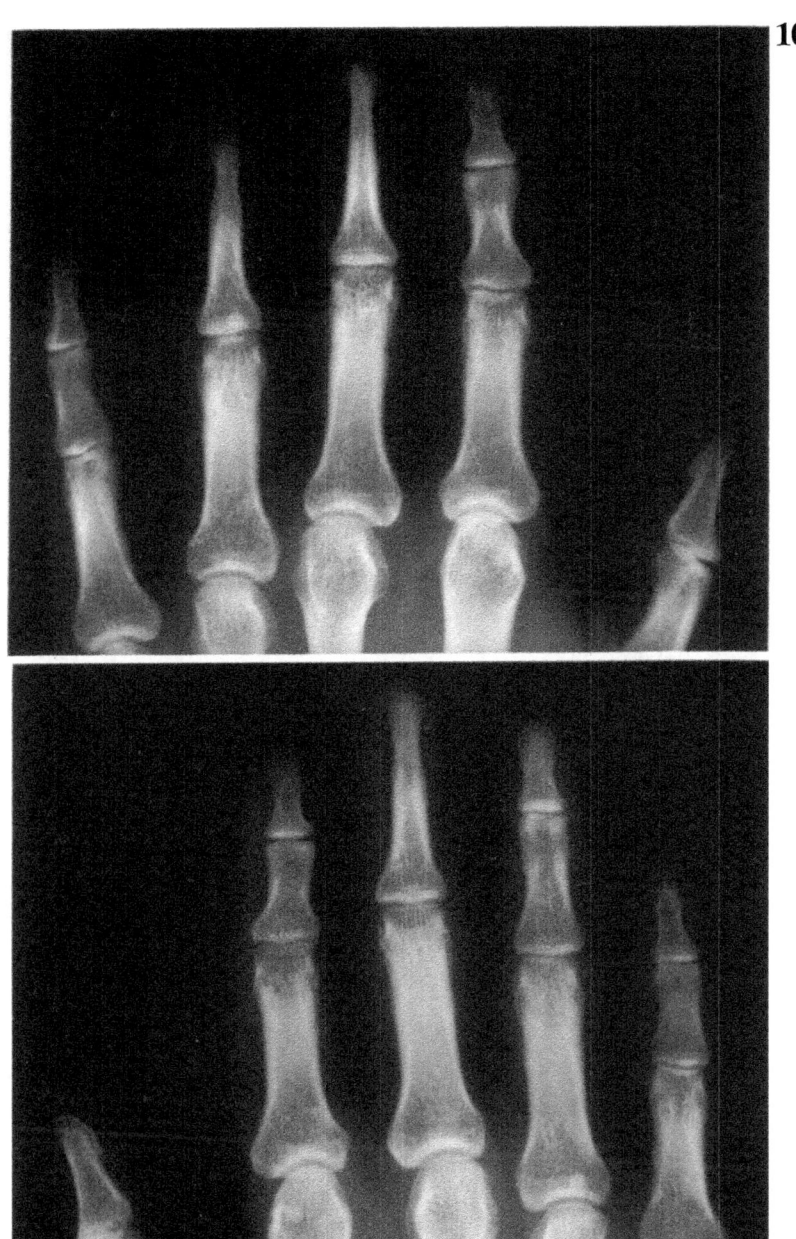

104

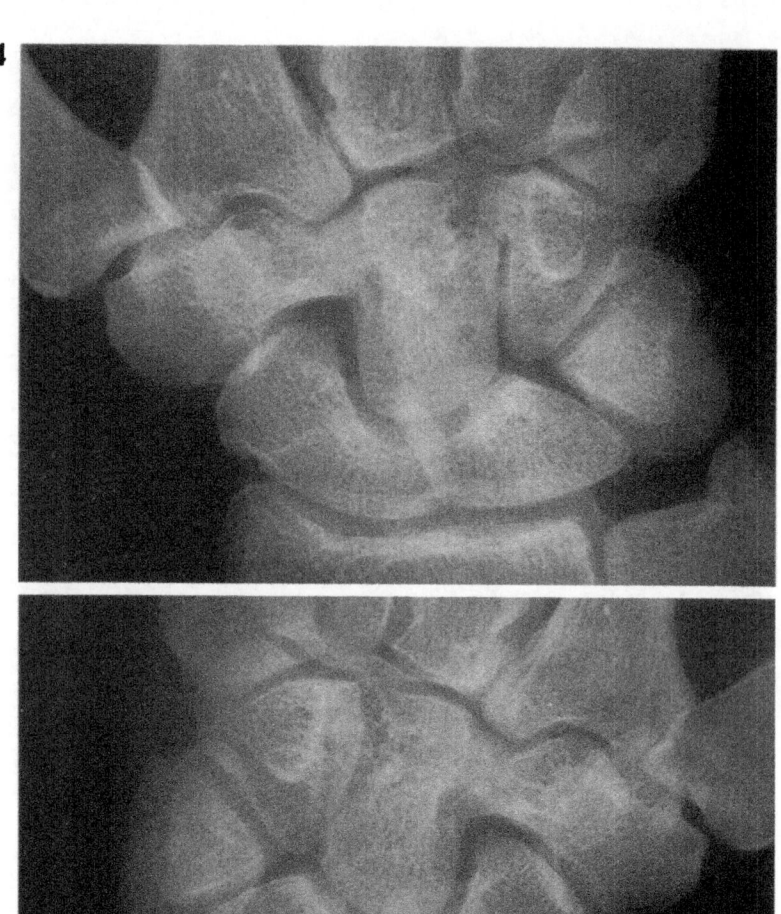

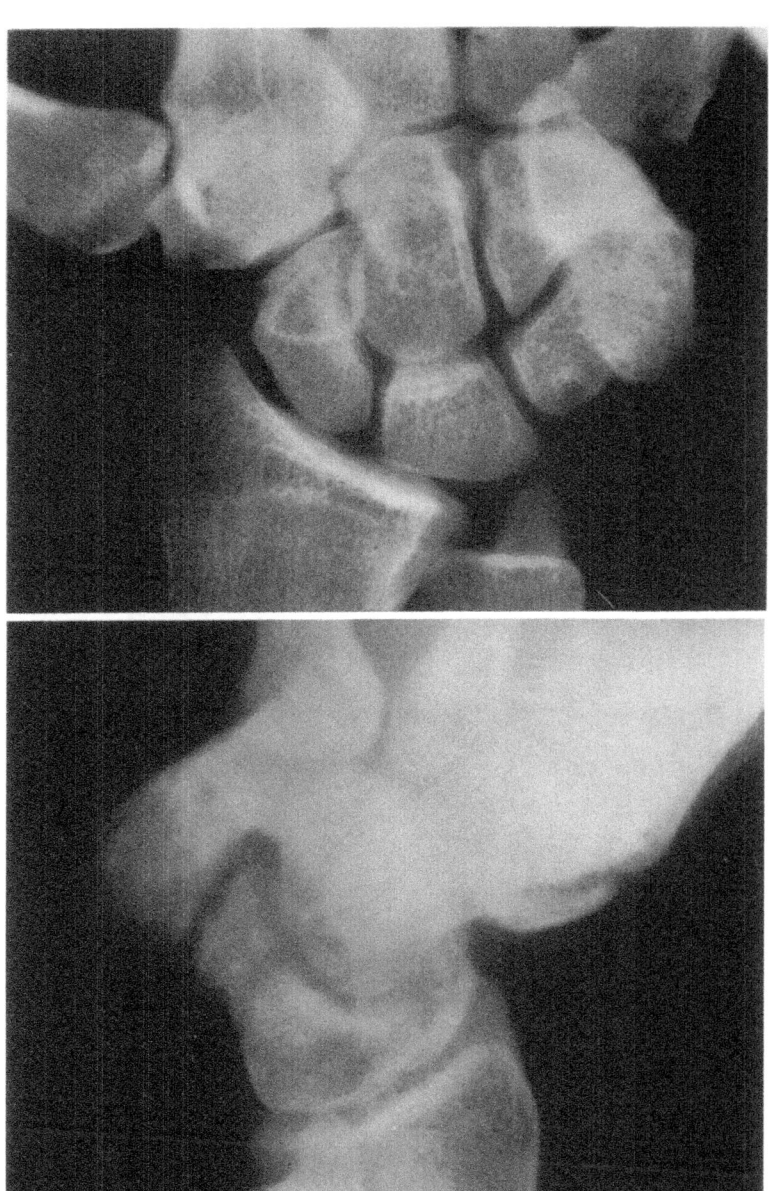

106

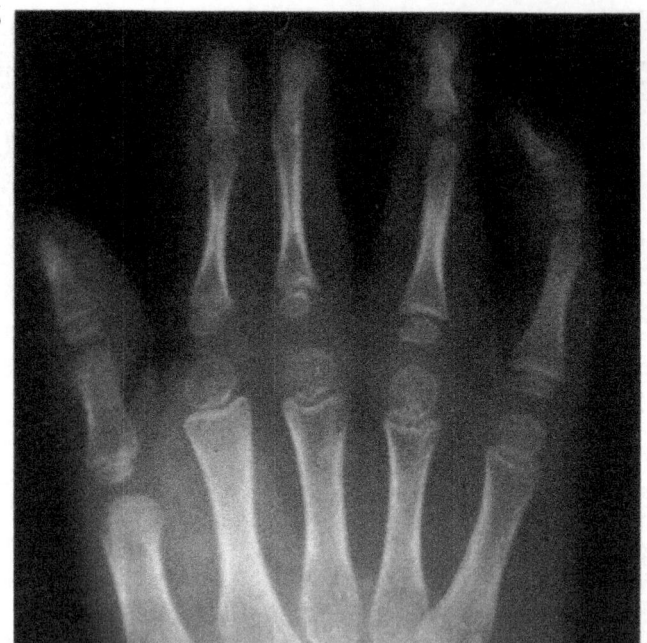

107

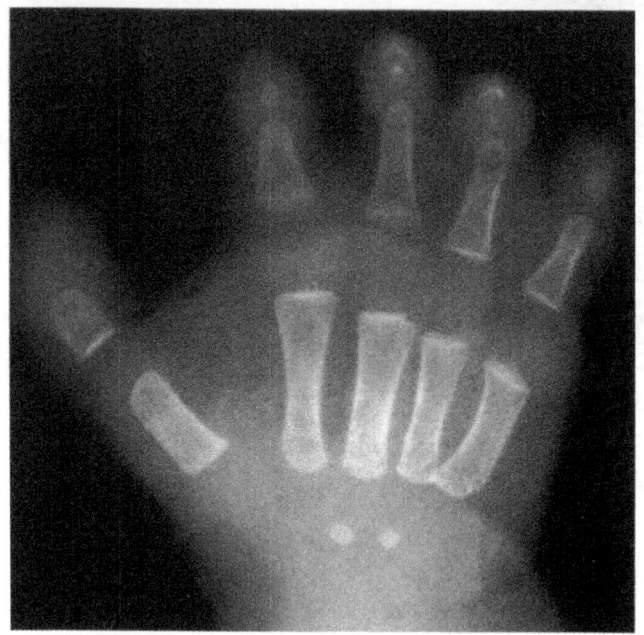

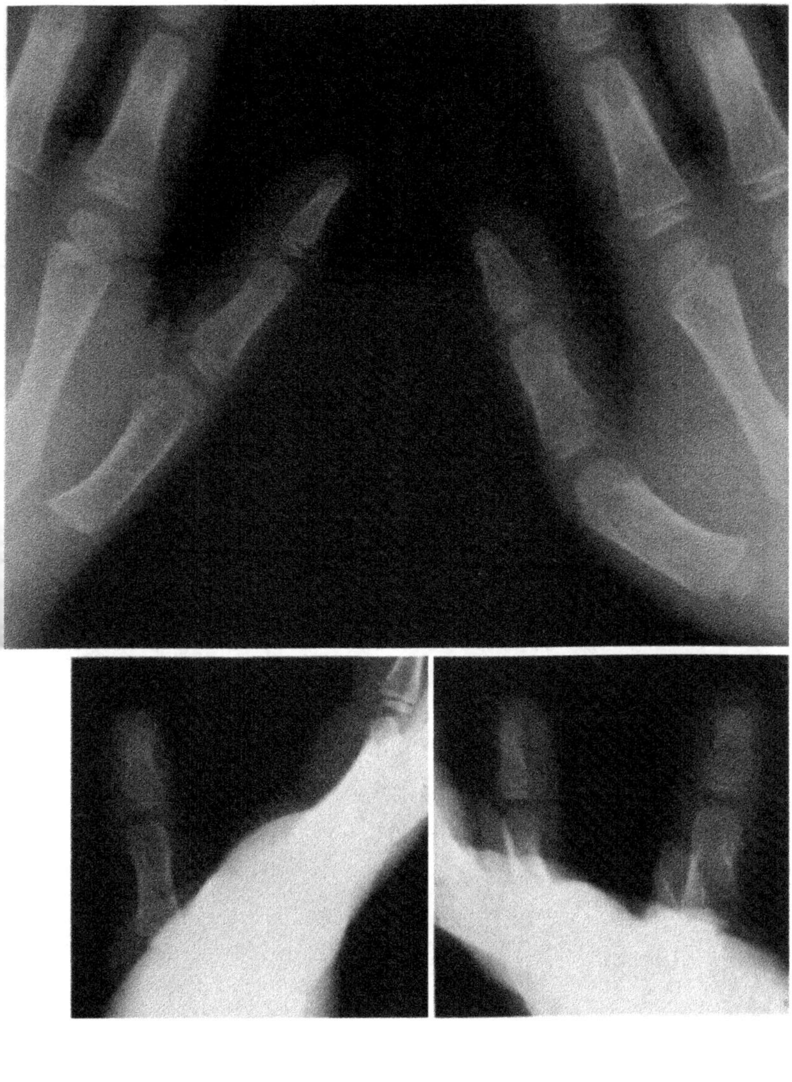

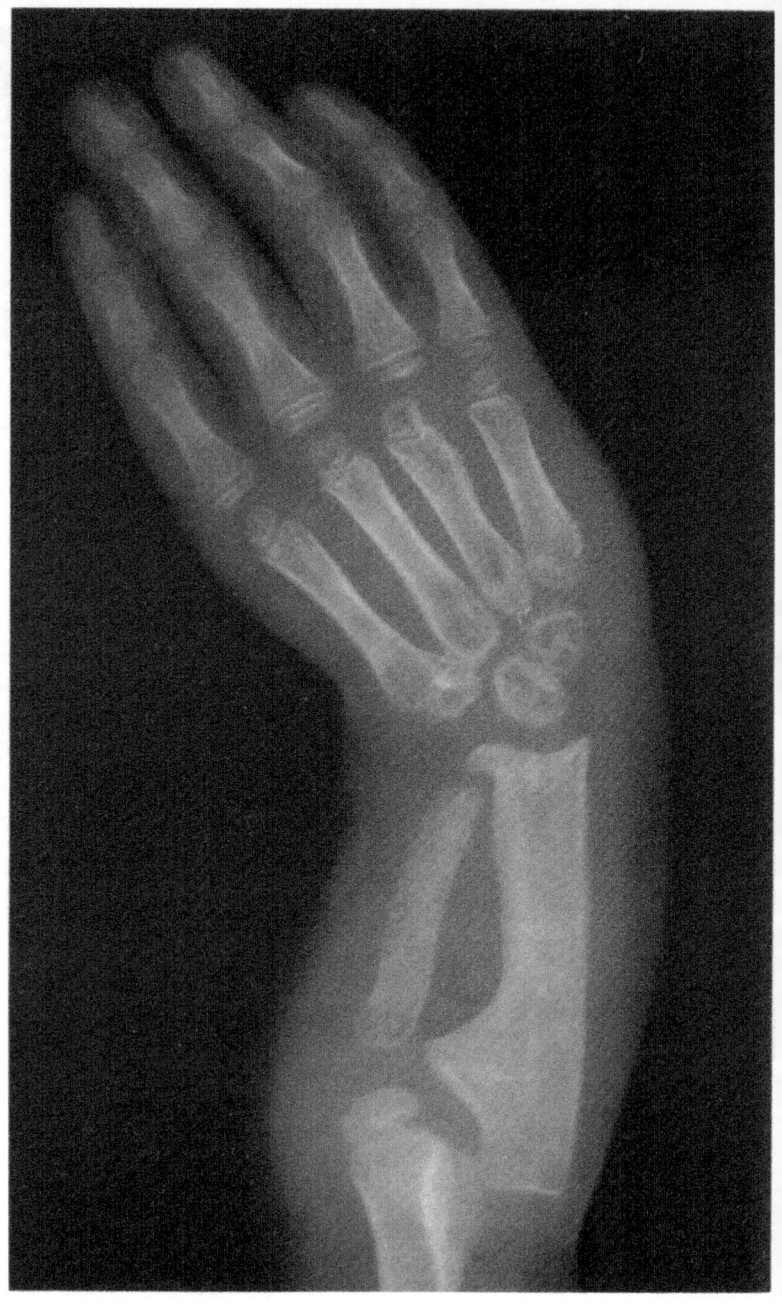

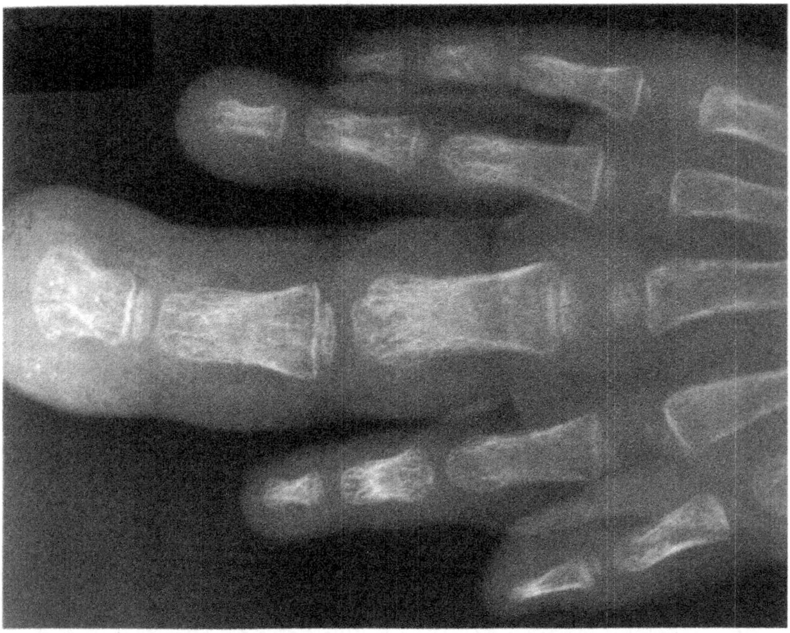

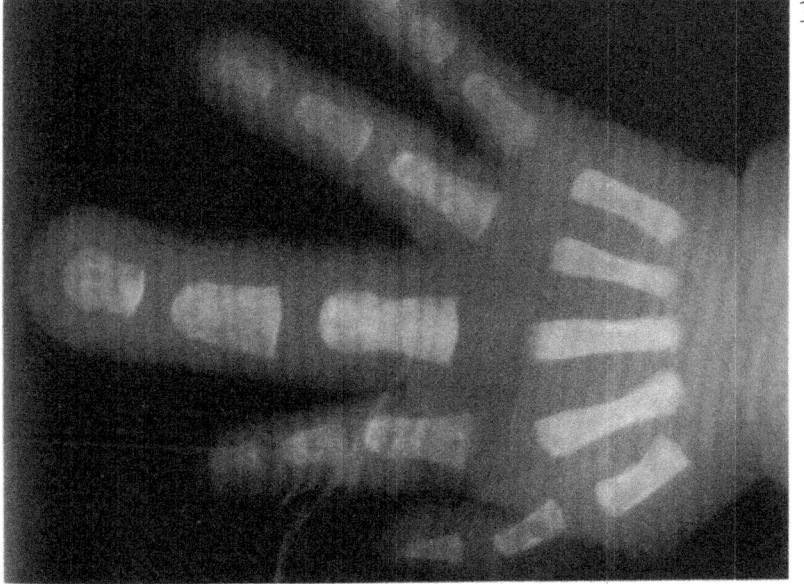

112

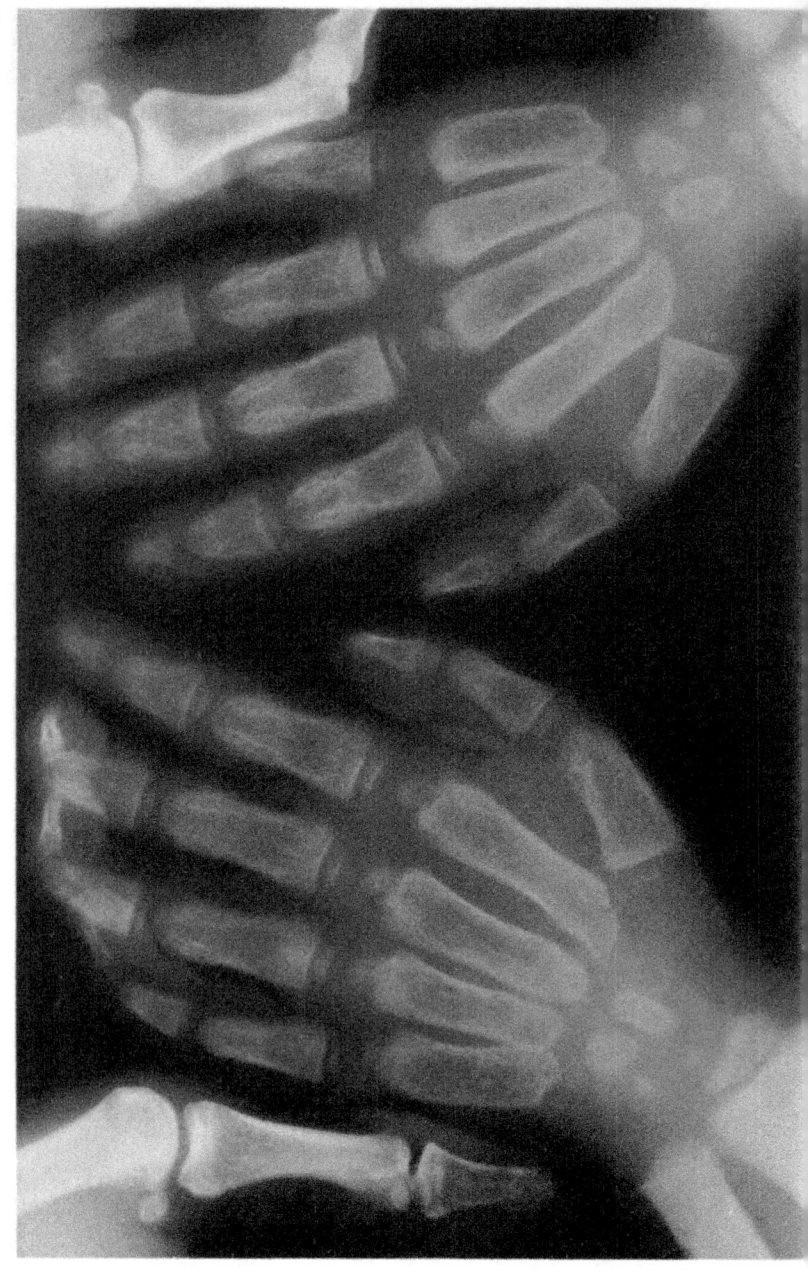

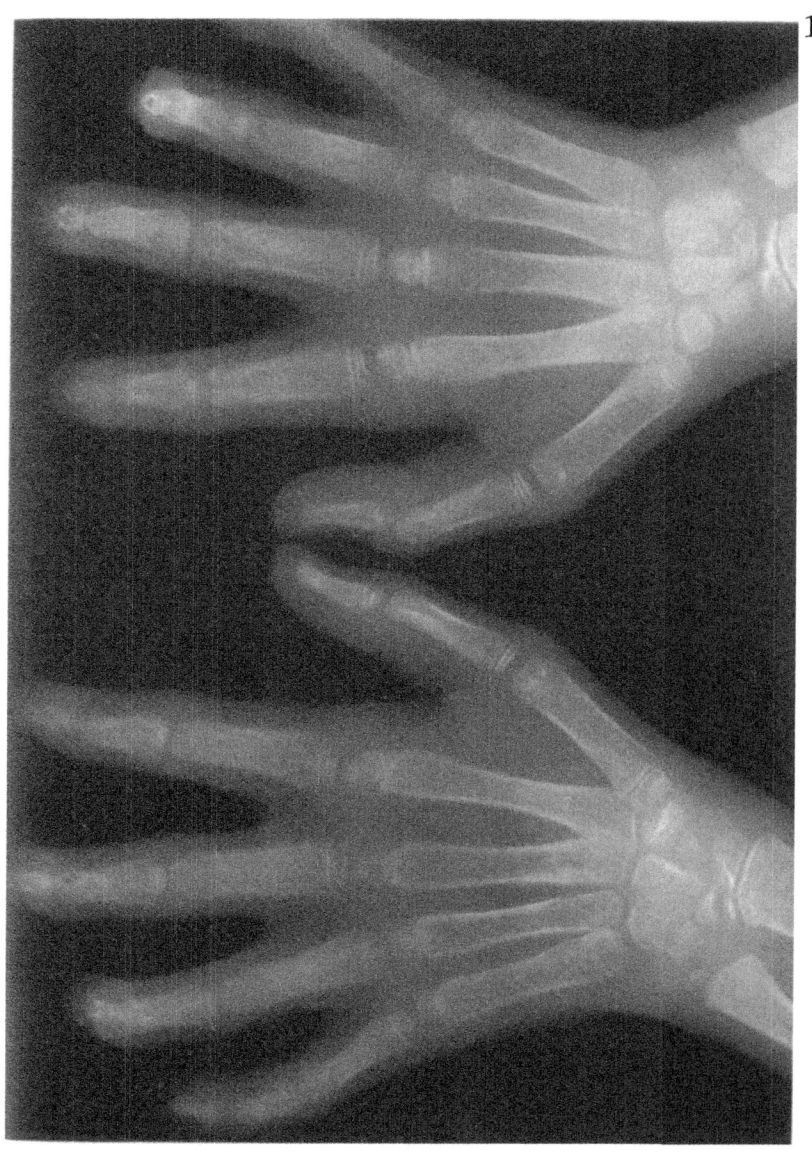

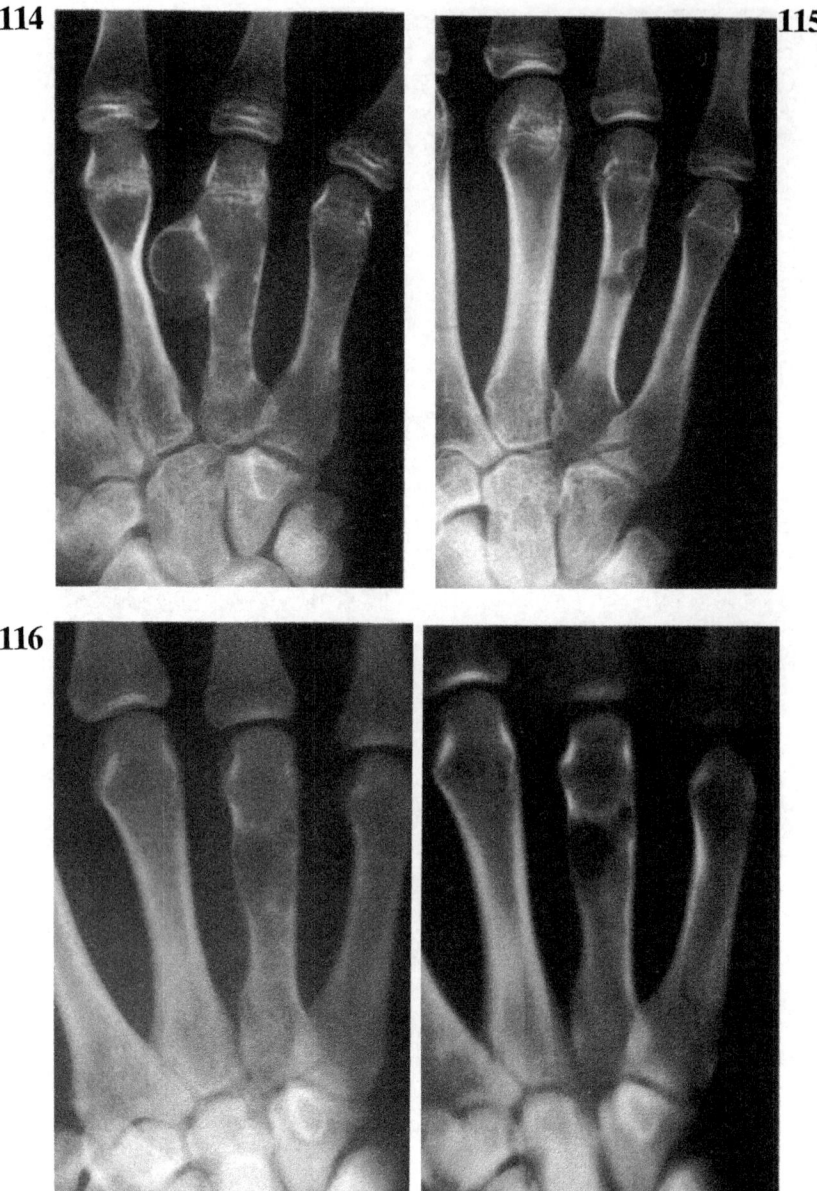

117

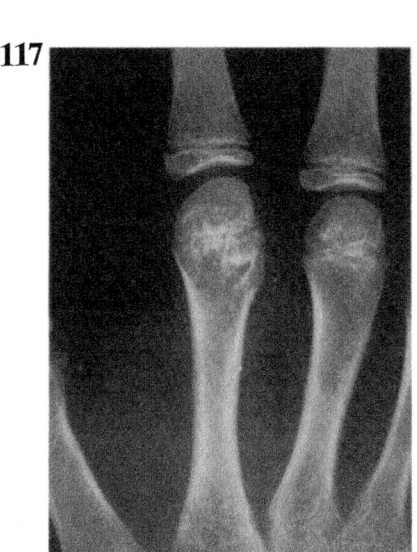

118

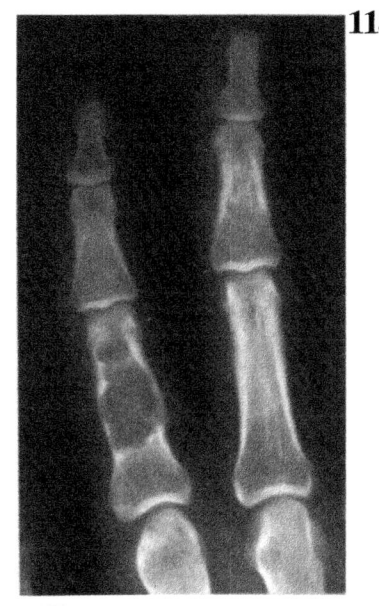

119

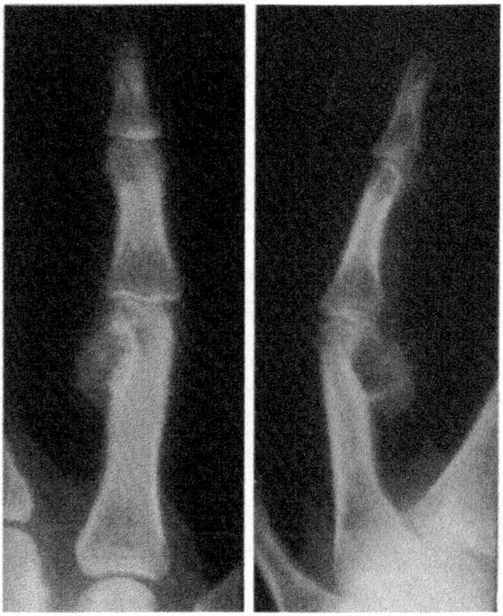

120

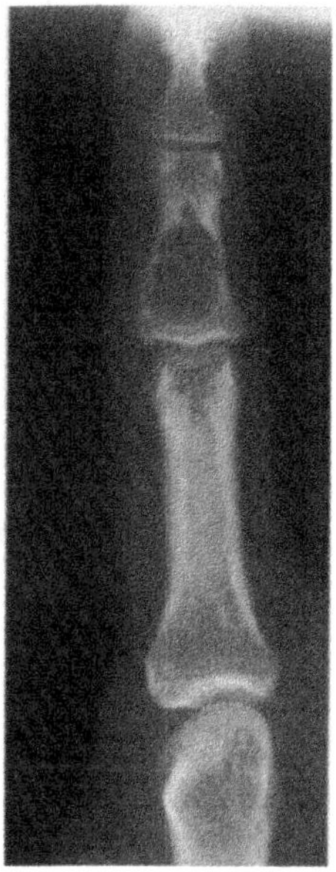

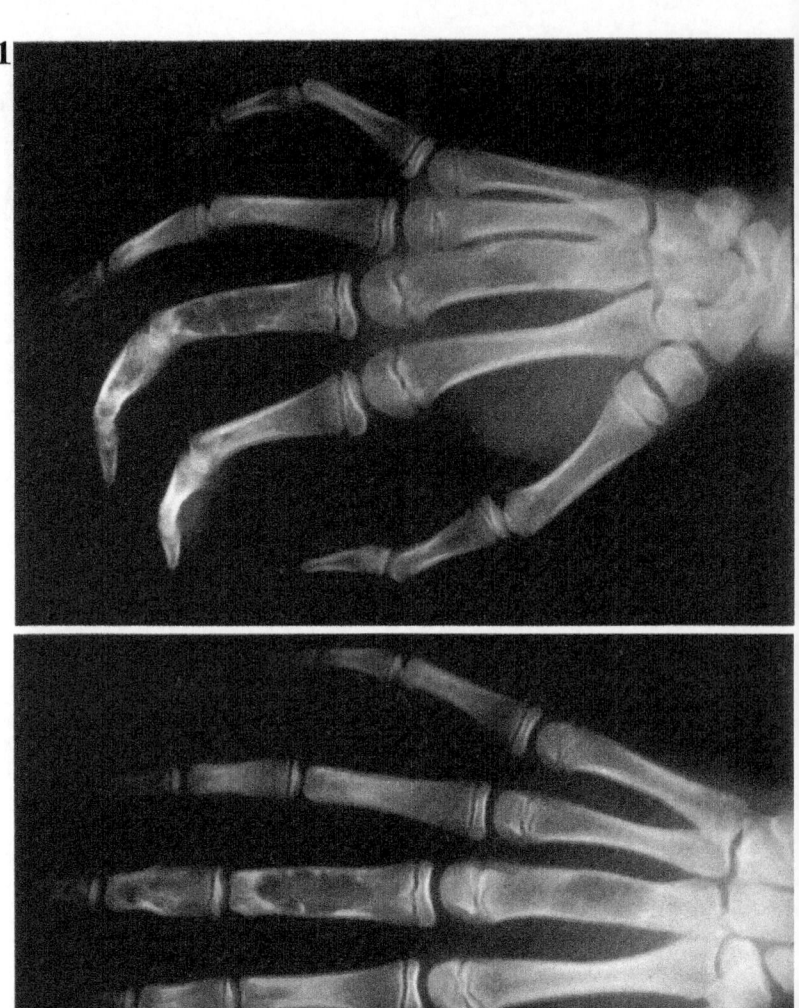

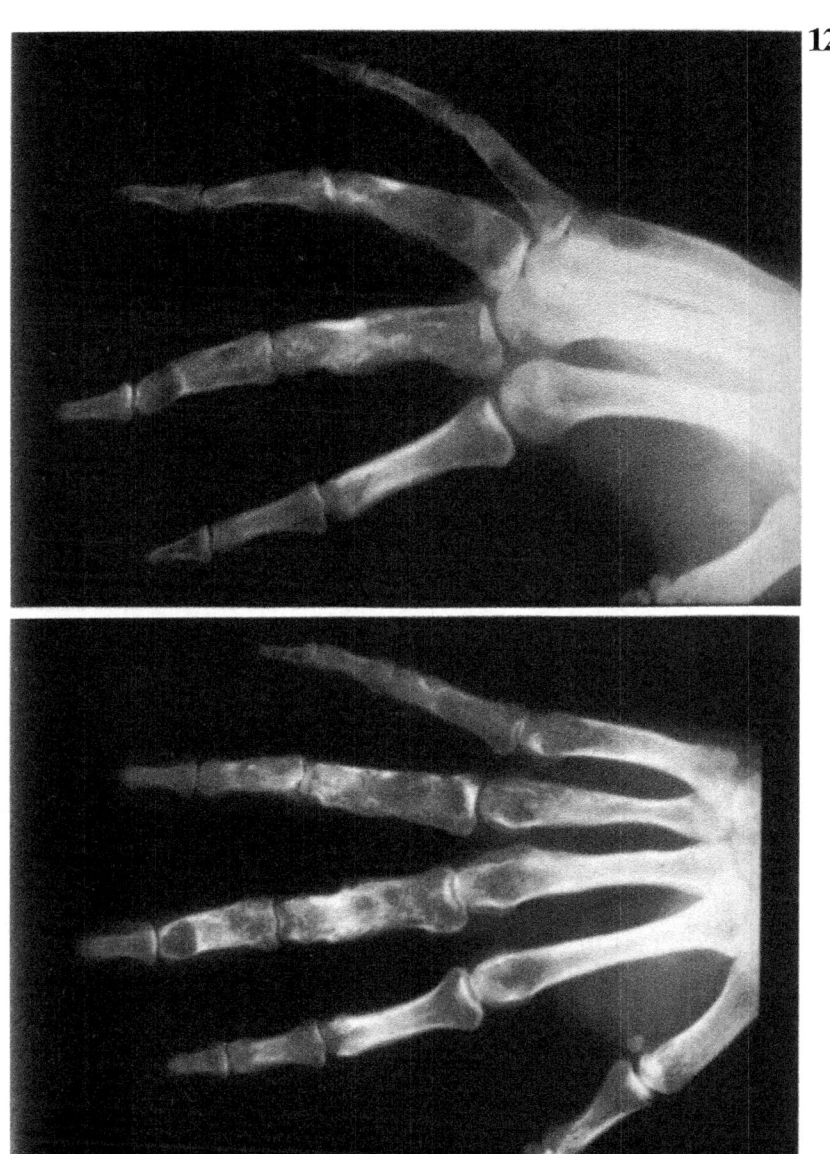

123

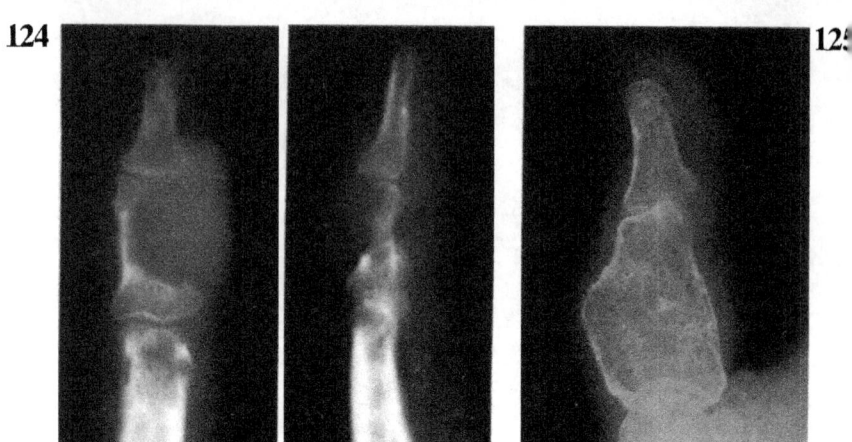

124

125

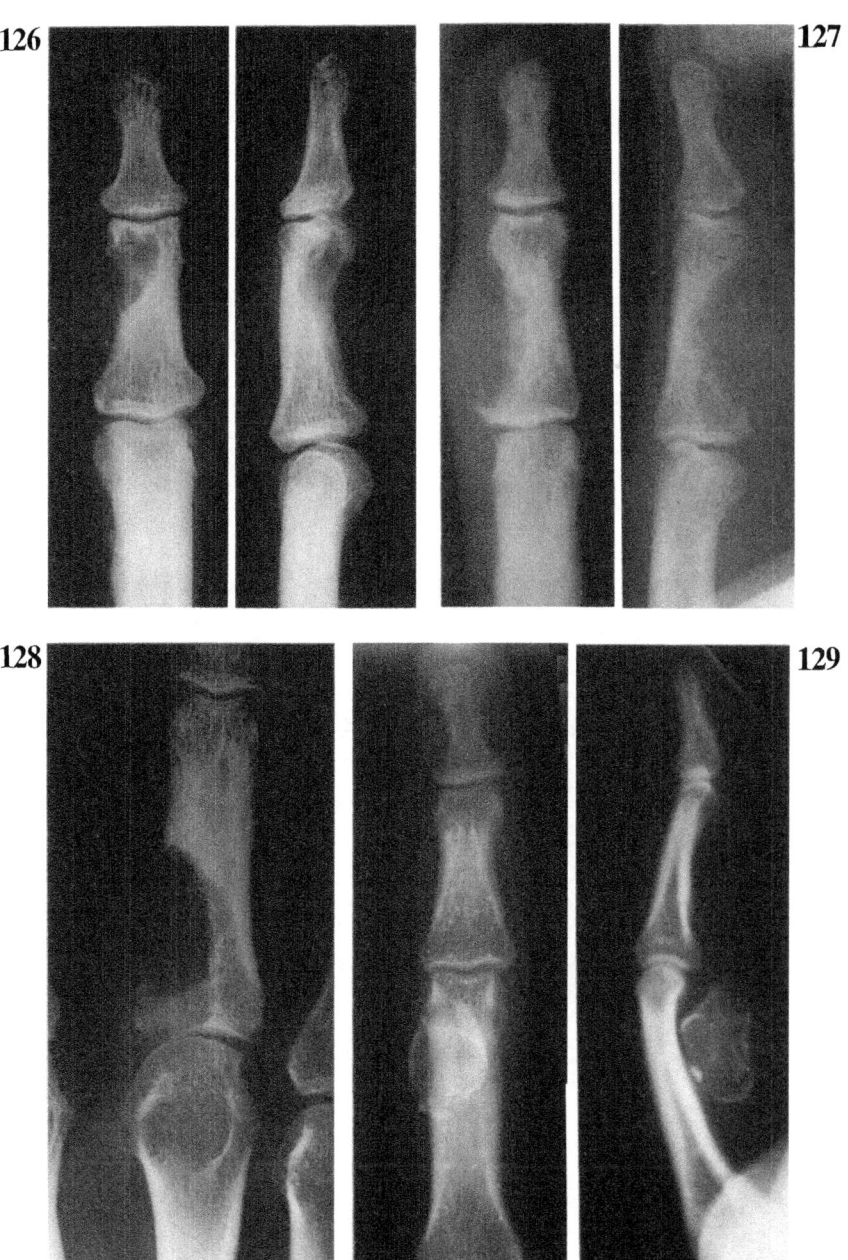

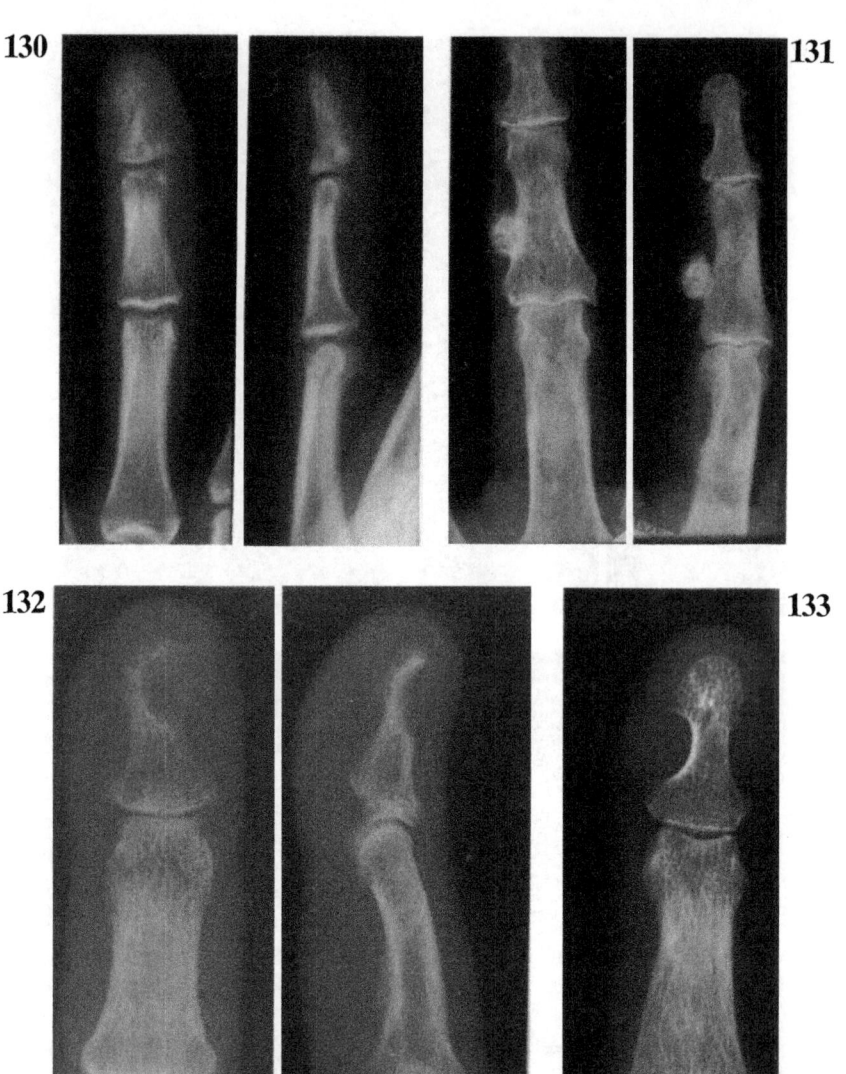

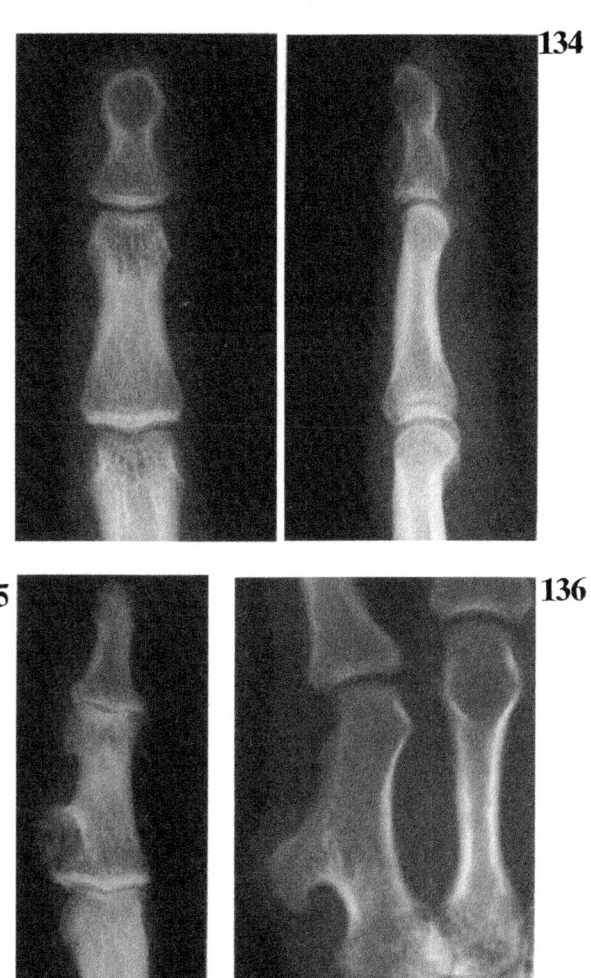

137

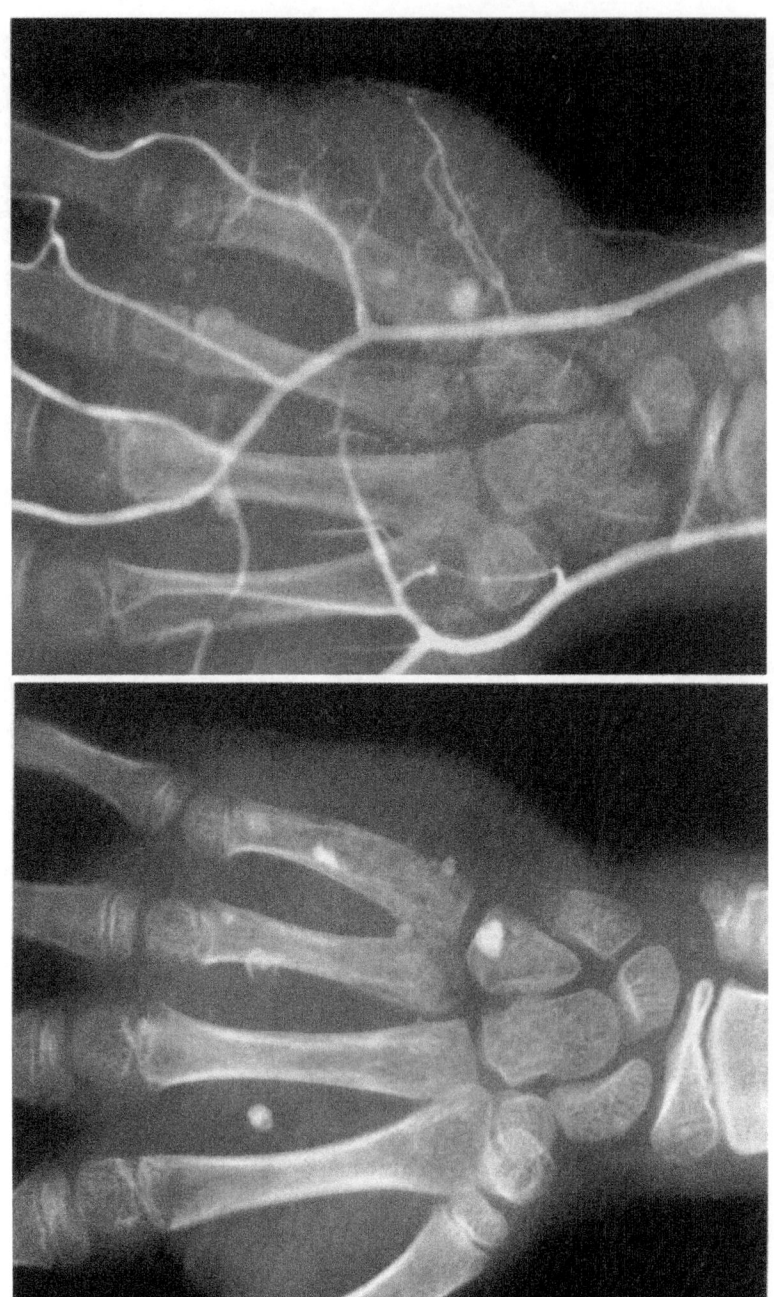

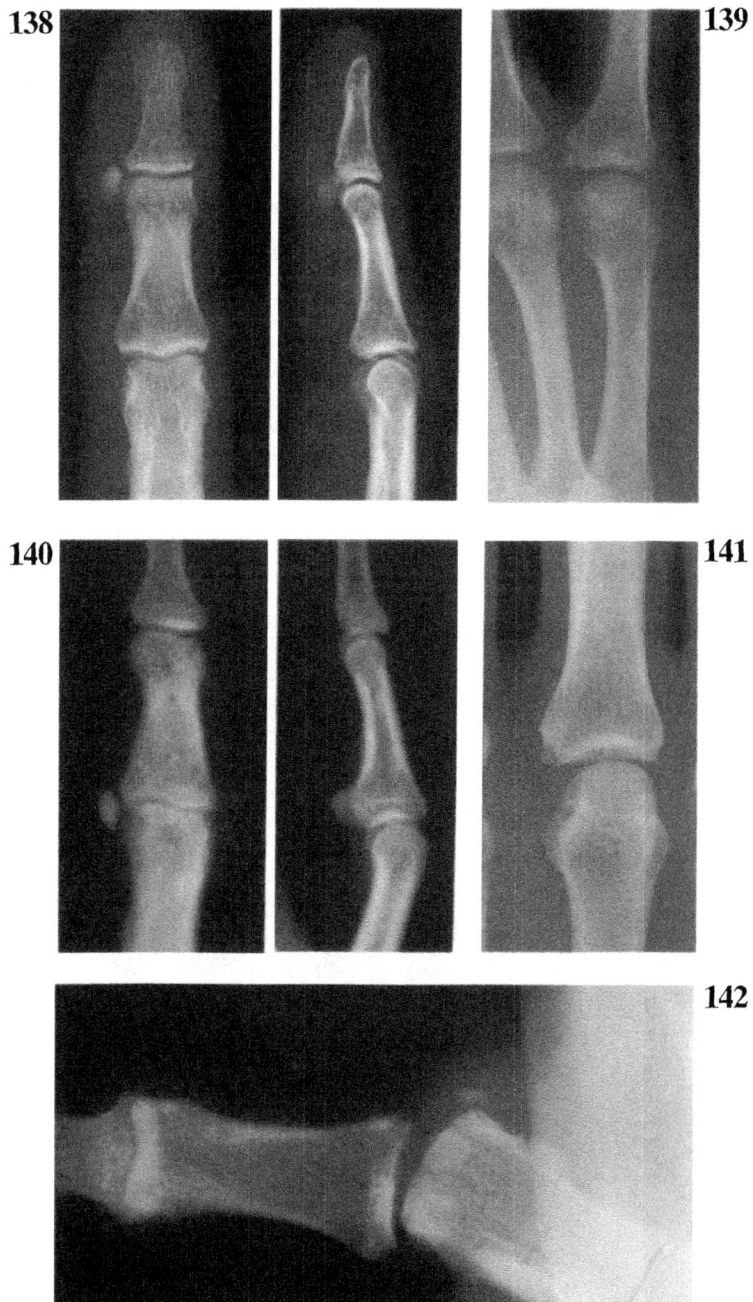

143

14

145

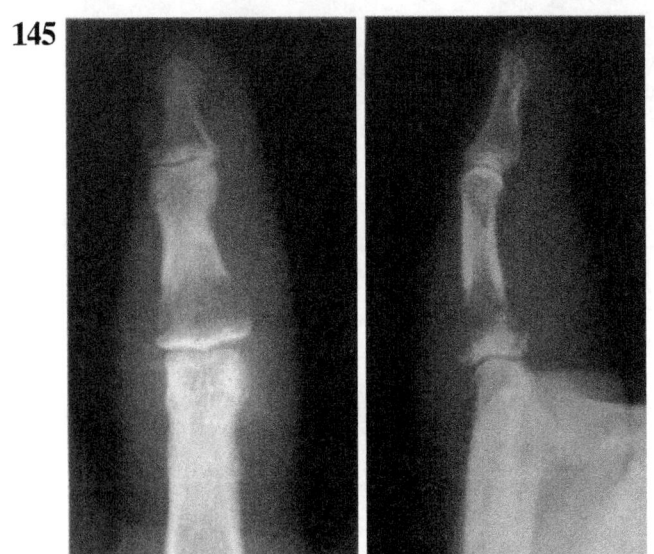

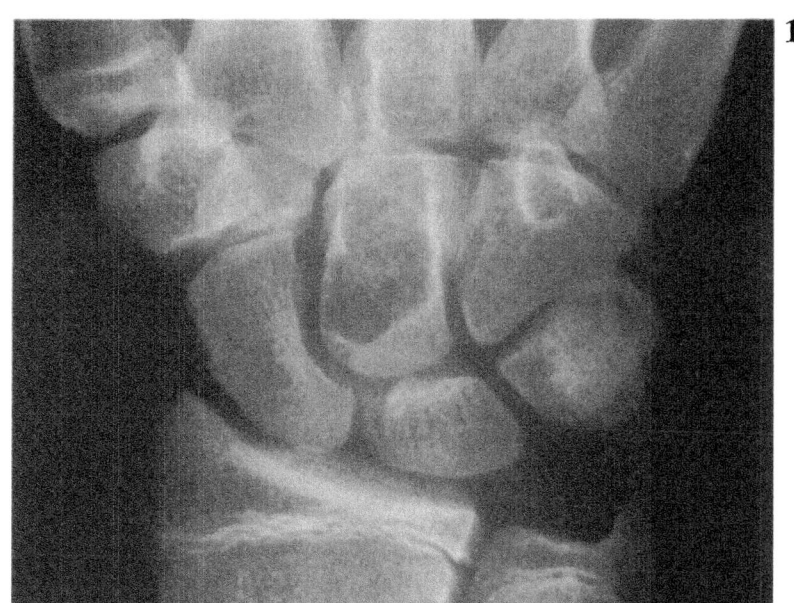

146

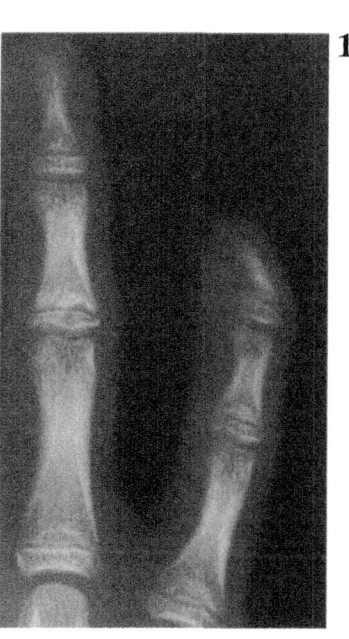

147

Part Two

Commentary with Corresponding Schemata

This frontal view of the hand is the view you will most often be asked to analyse. There are also other representations, which are more specific for regional studies: scaphoid, trapezium + base of the first metacarpal, cubital edge of the carpus and carpal tunnel.

The skeleton of the hand, carpus included, is composed of 27 main bone elements and of a variable number of accessory bone elements (sesamoids and accessory ossicles).

A good knowledge of some practical rules is necessary for a rapid analysis of the general harmony of the hand and of the size of the principal bone elements. *Anomalies in the length* of metacarpals and phalanges are rather frequent and often remain undetected when they

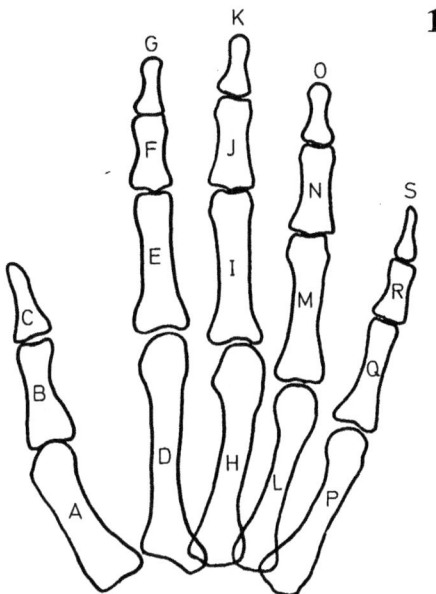

are unobtrusive. Since the length of the bones of the hand depends on size, biotype and sex, measurement tables with absolute values are of little interest. It is more profitable to consider dysharmony with regard to the opposite side and to the other bone elements.

The following practical rules should be kept in mind:
1. Decreasing length in the distal direction: metacarpal > proximal phalanx > middle phalanx > distal phalanx
2. The second metacarpal is the longest (*D*)
3. The longest phalanx is the proximal phalanx of the third finger (*I*)
4. The fourth metacarpal is the thinnest (*L*)
5. On the second and fifth fingers: proximal phalanx = middle phalanx + distal phalanx (E = F + G and Q = R + S)
6. On the fourth finger: metacarpal = proximal phalanx + distal phalanx (L = M + O)
7. On the fifth finger: metacarpal = proximal phalanx + middle phalanx (P = Q + R)
8. On the second and third fingers the sum of the lengths: metacarpal + proximal phalanx is identical (D + E = H + I)
9. First metacarpal = middle + distal phalanx of the fourth finger (A = N + O)
10. Proximal + distal phalanx of thumb = fifth metacarpal. Note that the distal phalanx of the thumb is longer than that of the other fingers. This is an important feature, since isolated shortening or brachytelephalangy of the thumb is relatively common.

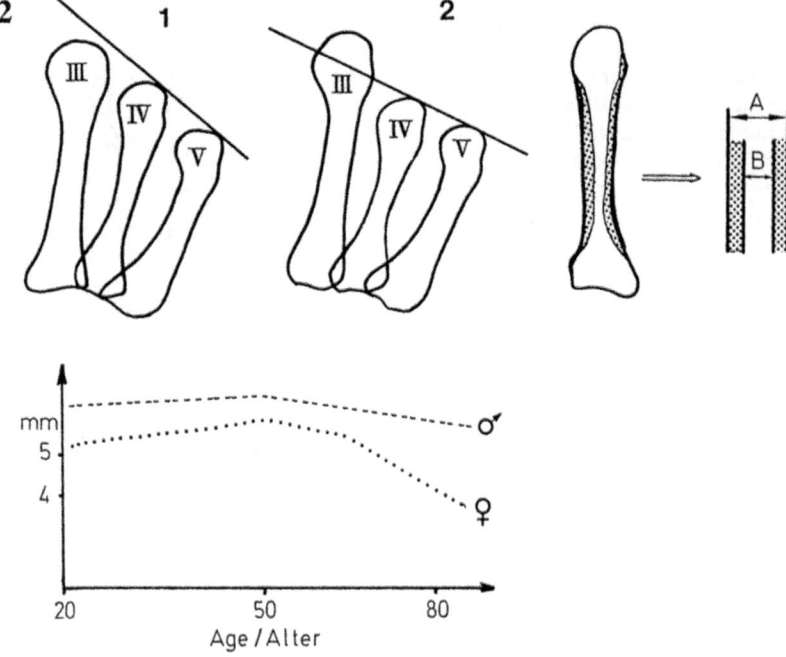

On a normal hand (*1*) the line tangential to the heads of the fifth and fourth metacarpals passes distal to the head of the third metacarpal. You can see this on the radiographic image. In the case of *shortening of the fourth metacarpal* (*2*) it intersects the head of the third; this is the brachymetacarpy of the fourth metacarpal of Archibald's metacarpal sign, which will be seen in different malformative syndromes, and more particularly in Turner's syndrome. The same situation also exists in the case of an abnormally lengthened third metacarpal, present only in Marfan's syndrome.

The cortical thickness of long bones diminishes with age. Measurement of cortical thickness at the midpoint of the second metacarpal constitutes a method for determining the degree of mineralization of the skeleton: cortical thickness = total diameter (A) – medullary thickness (B).

According to Garn's data, there is first an apposition phase increasing the total thickness, and then, after the age of 50 years, a phase of resorption which is much more rapid in females.

The carpal angle is formed by two lines, one tangential to the scaphoid and lunate, an the other tangential to the lunate and triquetrum. This angle is 131° ± 7° with the hand in the neutral position.

You will have to recognize characteristic decreases in the carpal angle in various malformative syndromes.

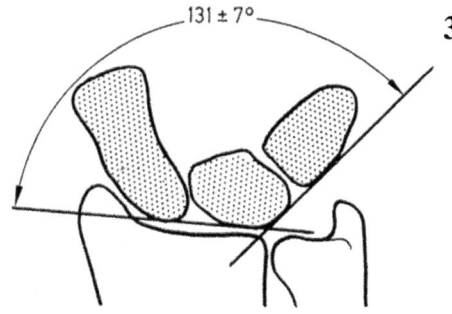

3

From a frontal view you must be able to recognize without hesitation the *bones of the carpus:*

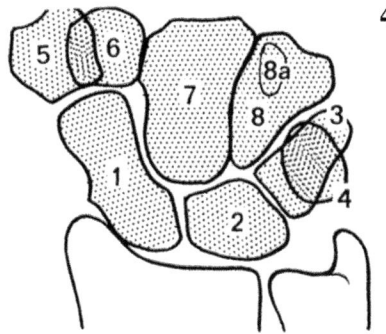

4

Proximal row:
1 Scaphoid
2 Lunate
3 Triquetrum
4 Pisiform, superimposed in its major part onto the triquetrum

Distal row:
5 Trapezium
6 Trapezoid, half superimposed onto the trapezium
7 Capitate
8 Hamate, with its hook (8a)

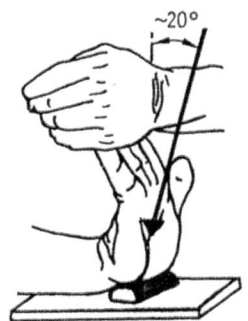

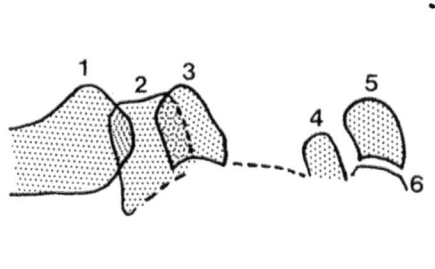

5

This particular *carpal tunnel view* (Incidence of Hart and Gaynor) is taken as indicated in the diagram. It visualizes:

On the radial aspect:
1 The base of the first metacarpal
2 The trapezium
3 The trapezoid

On the cubital aspect:
4 The hook of the hamate
5 The pisiform
6 The pisiform-triquetrum joint space

6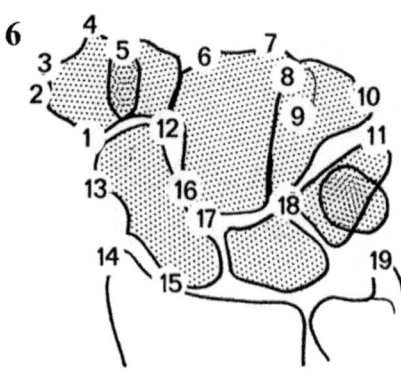

The accessory ossicles of the carpus are relatively rarely seen on radiographs (0.5%–2%). They are easily recognizable when they are projected onto a free edge or onto a joint space. Their occurrence is certainly underrated since they are often undetected on radiographs, especially when they are very small or when they are projected over a carpal bone. Certain small tendon calcifications can also be assimilated to the accessory ossicles.

According to Köhler, they are located as follows:

1 Epitrapezium
2 Calcification of the flexor carpi radialis
3 Paratrapezium or pretrapezium
4 Trapezium secundarium
5 Trapezoides secundarium
6 Os styloideum
7 Ossiculum Gruberi
8 Capitatum secundarium
9 Os hamuli proprium

10 Os vesalianum
11 Os ulnare externum
12 Os centrale carpi
13 Os radiale externum
14 Unfused ossification centre of the radial styloid process
15 Parascaphoid
16 Hypolunatum
17 Epilunatum
18 Epipyramis
19 Os triangulare

7

You will have identified here a small accessory ossicle (No. 3) = paratrapezium between the trapezium (*1*) and the base of the first metacarpal (*2*).

8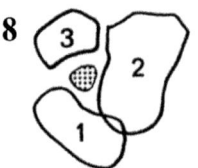

This os centrale carpi (No. 12) is more voluminous and located between the scaphoid (*1*), the capitate (*2*) and the trapezoid (*3*).

The os triangulare (No. 19) between the ulnar styloid process and the triquetrum is the most frequent accessory ossicle; it must thus be well known. It has variable form, size and site and may sometimes show bipartition. It must not be mistaken for an ancient traumatic avulsion of the ulnar styloid process, or for a calcified triangular 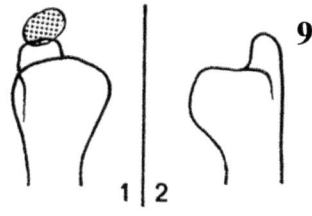 cartilage of the carpus. Arthrosic changes may render it unrecognizable.

Note her (*1*) the hypertrophic ulnar styloid process and the large os triangulare. Compare with the opposite side (*2*) where the ulnar styloid process is quite normal.

This os triangulare is located differently with regard to the ulnar styloid process and to the pisiform because of a slightly different position of the hand.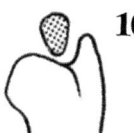

This other os triangulare is associated with an almost non-existent ulnar styloid process. Do not mistake it for an ancient traumatic avulsion. It is merely a normal variant.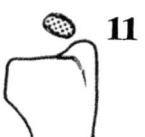

12

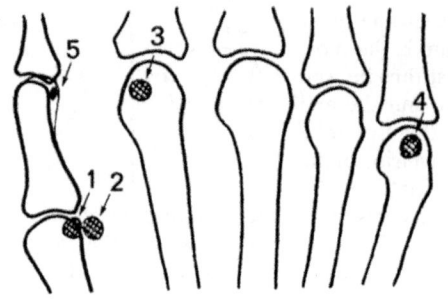

Sesamoid bones may occur within the tendons of the flexor digitorum (intratendinous sesamoids) or adjacent to the palmar aspect of the joints (periarticular sesamoids). They are projected over the metacarpal heads and the interphalangeal articulation of the thumb, and exceptionally elsewhere. The distribution of sesamoids is fairly constant:

Articulation	Number	Occurrence (%)
Metacarpophalangeal I	2	100
Metacarpophalangeal II	1	40
Metacarpophalangeal III	1	5
Metacarpophalangeal IV	1	2
Metacarpophalangeal V	1 or 2	75
Interphalangeal I	1 or 2	55
Interphalangeal proximal II–V	1	< 1
Interphalangeal distal II–V	1	< 1

Two sesamoids are permanent (*1* and *2*), medial and lateral to the metacarpophalangeal joint of the thumb. They appear at the age of 11 years in girls and at 13 years in boys, first the medial and then the lateral. Also very frequent, but not constant, are the sesamoids on the metacarpophalangeal joints of the second (*3*) and fifth (*4*) fingers and on the interphalangeal joint of the thumb (*5*).

The total number of sesamoids has no particular significance. They are slightly more frequent in males than in females. The size of the sesamoids increases in acromegalia; the sesamoid index of the thumb is defined as the product of its length and its width in millimetres. Normal values are about 25 in males and 20 in females, and they may range from 30 to 60 in acromegalia.

The metacarpals have *only one epiphysis* located at the proximal end on the thumb and at the distal end on the fingers. In this young patient you will easily recognize the epiphyses and the epiphyseal cartilage.

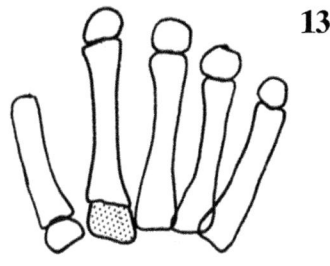

13

An additional epiphysis or *pseudoepiphysis* appears in the proximal part of the second metacarpal in about 10% of young people from 6 to 14 years of age, which should not be mistaken for a fracture. Pseudoepiphyses occurring in the phalanges are much more rare. They are usually transient and disappear before the end of the growth period.

The phalanges also have only one epiphysis; this is always proximal and has a flattened shape (*1*) with easily visible epiphyseal lines.

Cone-shaped-epiphyses (*2*) with their pointed tip extending towards the metaphysis, which shows a V-shaped indentation, can be seen in normal individuals aged 6–14 years, with a frequency of 2% in males and 7% in females. In normal subjects, cone epiphyses are oligophalangeal. On the contrary, multiple locations are pathognomonic of various dysostoses and dysplasiae (trichorhinophalangeal syndrome of Giedion, cleidocranial dysostosis, achondroplasia, etc.).

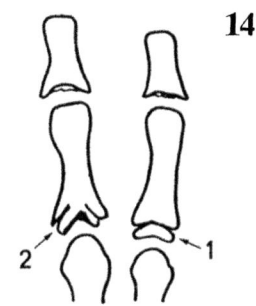

14

A focus of osteosclerosis is quite often seen on a bone of the hand; here, on the scaphoid bone. It is an area of increased density corresponding to compact bone, located in the spongiosa, either in its central part or adjacent to the cortex. It is a trivial disturbance of ossification .

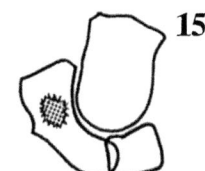

15

Sclerotic bone foci may occur anywhere; most commonly they involve the distal phalanges (cases 17 and 18), the metacarpals (case 19) and the capitate bone (case 16).

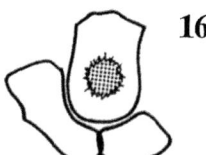

16

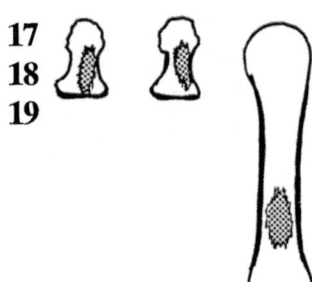

17
18
19

Since the cortex of the distal phalanges is very thin, the sclerotic foci are often peripheral.

Note the unsharp limits of the increased density area in the spongiosa of this metacarpal bone.

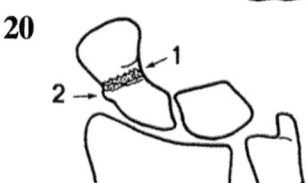

20

This *fracture of the scaphoid* is easily recognizable by (*1*) the transverse and irregular translucency across the bone. The overlapping on the radial edge (*2*) does not correspond to displaced fragments but to the crest which always, at this level, forms the limit between the neck and the body of the bone.

Of carpal bone fractures, 85% involve the scaphoid; 70% of them are located on the scaphoid neck, a somewhat narrowed segment corresponding roughly to the middle part of the bone. Distal fractures of the tubercle or fractures of the proximal pole are much rarer. Displacement of the fragments is uncommon. In the case of marked displacement, the fracture is usually associated with retrolunate luxation of the carpal bone. The proximal fragment is more fragile since it has limited blood supply. Pseudarthrosis and necrosis of the proximal fragment are commoner the more proximal the fracture is located.

It is incorrect to believe that a scaphoid fracture can remain undetected by X-rays. This occurs in only about 2% of cases. Pain on palpation is very characteristic; supplemental views with different positioning of the carpus and different inclination of the beam may be necessary to aid in diagnosing the fracture.

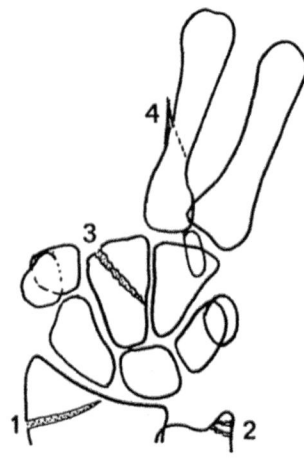

21

This traumatism by crushing is responsible for *several fractures:*

1 Fracture of the radial styloid process extending to the radiocarpal joint
2 Fracture of the ulnar styloid process
3 Oblique fracture of the capitate bone
4 Spiroid fracture of the diaphysis of the fourth metacarpal

Fracture of the capitate bone is uncommon and usually results from a compression process.

126

The trapezium – base of the thumb metacarpal area is a frequent site for fractures but more rarely for dislocations. Note here the disalignment in the radial edge of the carpus with displacement of the trapezium in the radial direction. This is a *fracture dislocation of the trapezium.* The fracture line proper is not visible; its demonstration requires supplemental radiographs, eventually tomograms. The difficulty of isolating the trapezium on X-rays accounts for the quite frequent failure to diagnose traumatic lesions of this bone.

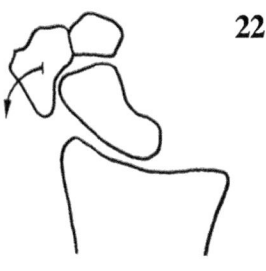

22

This fracture (1) at the base of the thumb metacarpal with displacement of the distal fragment and overriding (2) is readily recognizable. The fracture is extra-articular. The second variety of fracture occurring at this site is Bennett's fracture, an oblique articular fracture displacing the medial fragment of the metacarpal base. This fragment can be small when there is a simple fracture of the beak of the first metacarpal without displacement; it can therefore easily pass undetected. Sometimes, on the contrary, the whole metacarpal is pulled upwards and laterally, due to the pull of the abductor pollicus longus. A third variety of fracture is Rolando's fracture, a comminuted fracture of the epiphysis with dislocation of the trapezometacarpal joint.

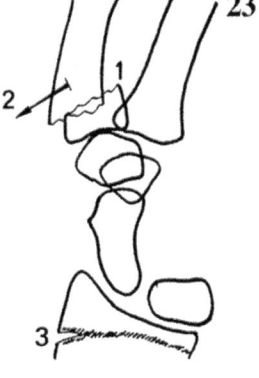

23

On this same radiograph, you will not have of course mistaken for a fracture the linear translucency delineated by the dense line of the radial metaphysis (3), corresponding in this adolescent to remains of epiphyseal lines.

24

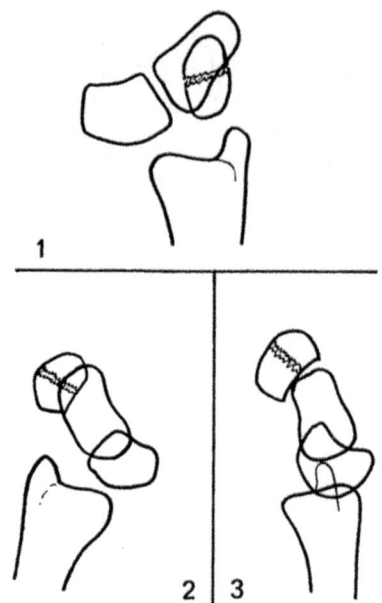

This *fracture of the pisiform bone* is but faintly visualized on a classical frontal X-ray of the carpus (*1*). When there is any definite post-traumatic pain, suitable radiographic investigations must be performed, and for the chosen incidence several radiographs must be taken with various positionings.

Thus, this fracture is much better visualized on the two radiographs (Garraud's view) (*2*) with the hand in semi-supination, and then with maximal extension of the wrist (*3*).

Fracture of the pisiform is not very common; it results from a fall on the palmar side of the wrist in hyperextension.

25

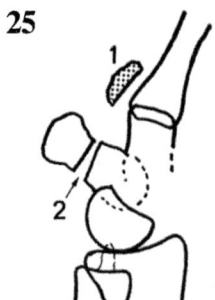
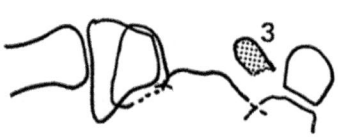

The fracture of the hook of the hamate is classic (tennis, golf), but its diagnosis is difficult.

The hook of the hamate is projected onto a cutaneous point where its palpation is relatively difficult, situated 1.5 cm from the pisiform, on a line joining the pisiform to the head of the third metacarpal.

The radiological diagnosis of the fracture of the hook of the hamate is also difficult; tomographs are often necessary since in many injured patients the carpal canal view of Hart and Gaynor (see case 5) cannot be performed since the positioning is too painful. Moreover, in Garraud's projection, the hook of the hamate is often superimposed onto the base of the fifth metacarpal.

Garraud's projection shows here a lateral view (*1*), Hart and Gaynor's projection an axial view (*3*) of the ruptured hook of hamate. The pisotriquetral joint (*2*) is easily visible here with abnormal widening on the proximal side, corresponding to subluxation of the pisiform.

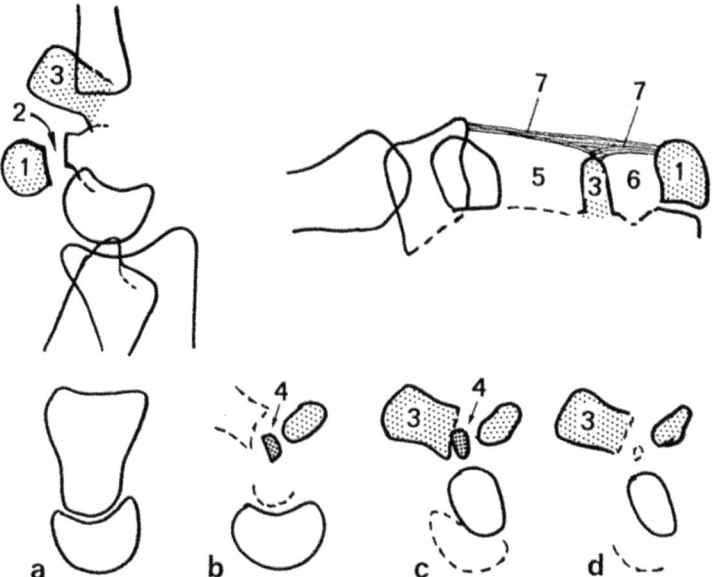

26

On this frontal view of the wrist you will have, correctly, noted the absence of abnormality.

This radiograph taken with the hand in Garraud's position shows clearly the displacement of the pisiform (*1*) and the significantly enlarged pisotriquetral joint (*2*). The hook of the hamate (*3*) seems normal, however.

This is a very classic pitfall. In fact, *fractures of the hamate,* and particularly those occurring through the base of the hamulus, may result from a mild trauma. Standard frontal and lateral radiographs are normal. Often the diagnosis is made, from *the tomograms,* only a few months later when there are complications such as persistent pain, carpal tunnel syndrome or ulnar nerve palsy. Lateral tomograms are the most informative.

Here you will note:
– Section *a* (lunate – capitate): normal
– Sections *b* (lunate – hamate), *c* and *d* (triquetral – hamate): fracture of the hamate with detachment of the hook of the hamate (*3*) and central sequestrum (*4*)

Let us recall here the strategic position of the hook of the hamate (*3*): it separates the carpal tunnel proper (*5*) from the ulnar carpal tunnel or canal of Guyon (*6*) between the hamulus (*3*) and the pisiform (*1*). The hook also serves as the distal anchor for the ulnar margin of the transverse carpal ligament (*7*).

The hook of the hamate develops independently of the body of the hamate; fusion occurs at the age of 15 years. Failure of fusion is uncommon; when present it is responsible for the os hamuli proprium (cf. case 6: accessory ossicle No. 9), which has smooth and corticated margins and is thus easy to differentiate from an avulsion fracture.

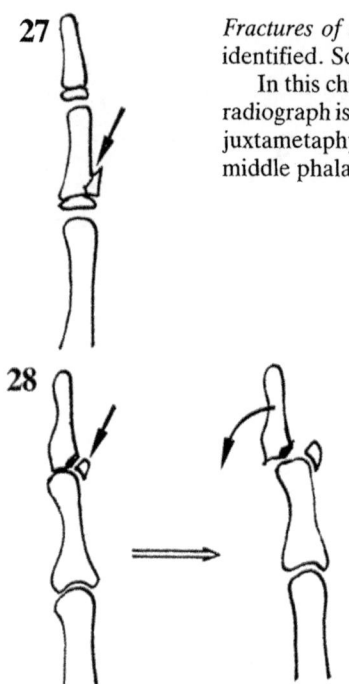

27 *Fractures of the metacarpals and phalanges* are usually readily identified. Sometimes, however, diagnosis is not so evident.

In this child with persistent epiphyseal cartilage, the frontal radiograph is normal. Only a lateral view enables us to identify a juxtametaphyseal disalignment in the dorsal aspect of the middle phalanx, corresponding to a small avulsion fracture.

28

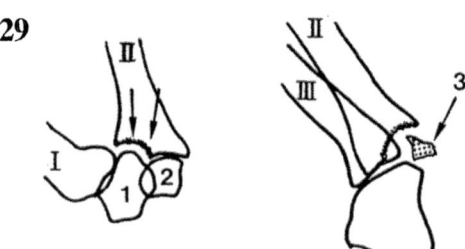

Mallet finger

It is the same in the case of this adult. Only the lateral view visualizes the avulsion of the dorsal part of the base of the distal phalanx. This articular fracture is in fact an osteotendinous avulsion of the distal insertion of the extensor digitorum.

Note, however, the absence of subluxation during flexion responsible for the mallet finger deformity. The major risk is ankylosis.

29

On this frontal view you will recognize a peculiar "indentation" on the radial aspect of the base of the second metacarpal which seems to articulate with the trapezium (*1*) anteriorly to the trapezoid (*2*). This image is never seen in normal conditions.

It is, however, very difficult to prove the traumatic nature of this anomaly. Only a special view, the so-called "hunch-backed carpus" view, showed the basal fragment of this undetected fracture (*3*). In fact, the patient came to the X-ray department because of chronic pain evoking rhizarthrosis of the thumb.

For traumatisms of the hand, a general rule should be remembered: the clinician should not send the patient for a "frontal and lateral radiograph of the hand" but should rather ask for a "radiographic investigation to search for a fracture, with the necessary special views"; as to the radiologist, he or she must adapt the projections with regard to the localization of the pain, and eventually take the initiative in performing tomograms.

Diaphyseal fractures of metacarpals and phalanges are usually spiroid or oblique transversally. This *longitudinal greenstick fracture,* with several fracture lines, of the proximal phalanx of the third finger was caused by crushing and not, as the majority of fractures, by hyperflexion or extension movements.

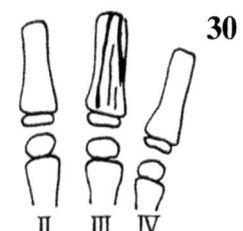

30

II   III   IV

A characteristic traumatic lesion in children is the *epiphyseal separation.* This lesion is often recognized only after weeks or even months when there is already periosteal reaction, or rather hyperostosis on periosteal separation.

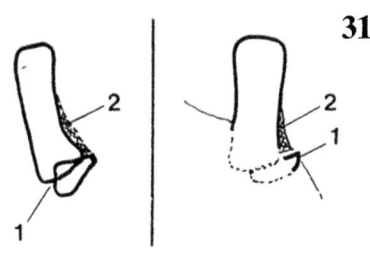

31

Do not forget that on a frontal radiograph of the hand the thumb is seen obliquely. Note on this view, as well as on a true frontal view in hyperpronation:

1 Disalignment between the epiphysis and diaphysis
2 New bone formation corresponding to the periosteal reaction

Metacarpophalangeal dislocation of the thumb is commonly seen in sports (skiing) and professional injuries. It is seldom seen on X-rays because it is often replaced spontaneously. The patient complains about persistent pain due to instability of the thumb and, thus, markedly diminished muscular strength. The radiograph, however, is negative!

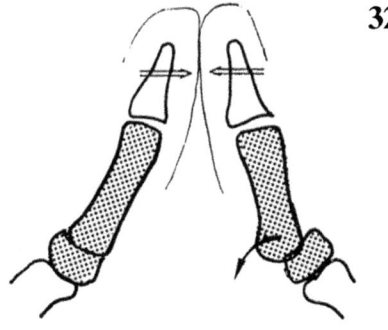

32

Dislocation is of course only possible when there is avulsion and/or elongation of the ligaments. The major risk is relatively rapidly occurring arthrosis. Eaton's technique, which we have used here, is a *stress radiograph.* The patient presses his or her thumbs against each other in order to produce the dislocation, which will be evaluated by comparison with the normal side. Such a manoeuvre, however, entails some risks: displacement of fragments of an unrecognized fracture (Bennett's fracture or fracture of the trapezium) and tendinoligamentous interposition, called Stener's effect. A stress radiograph should only be performed when demanded by the surgeon, when there is a definite clinical suspicion, and then with the patient under block anaesthesia.

33

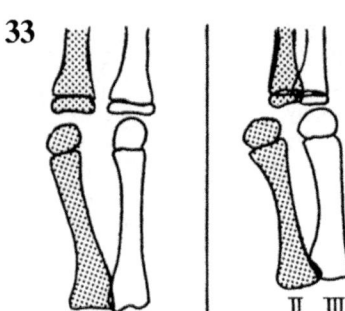

II III   II III

Metacarpophalangeal or interphalangeal dislocation is often more evident clinically than radiographically.

On this oblique projection you will have certainly readily made the diagnosis of metacarpophalangeal dislocation of the second finger. On a frontal view the disalignment is much less marked. It is less important to make the diagnosis of dislocation than to rule out an associated fracture which might be overlooked since the only clue is often only a small bone fragment at the base of a phalanx.

34

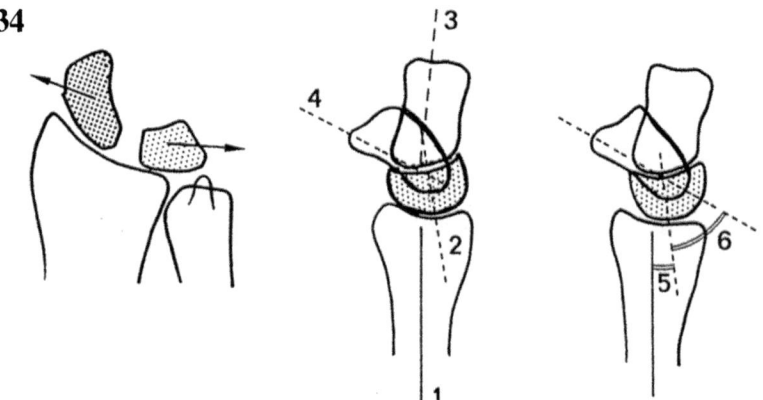

This frontal radiograph shows a very clear scapholunate gap or diastasis of about 5 mm, quite an abnormal configuration. We will now deal with the very difficult problem of *instabilities of the wrist*. The scapholunate joint is of primary importance in the biomechanics of the wrist. Ligamentous injury followed by scapholunate subluxation is one of the multiple causes of wrist instability. This pathology is probably very common, but it is doubtlessly often unrecognized because of the complexity and lack of precision of radiological measurements.

On a lateral radiograph in the neutral position, the following lines should be traced:

− The axis of the radius (*1*)
− The axis of the lunate (*2*): perpendicular through the centre of a line joining the anterior and posterior horn of the lunate, always readily visible
− The axis of the capitate (*3*): line joining the midpoint of the proximal convexity with the midpoint of the base of the third metacarpal
− The axis of the scaphoid (*4*): line joining the distal and proximal convex extremities of the bone
− The radiolunate angle (*5*): angle formed by (*1*) and (*2*)
− The scapholunate angle (*6*): angle formed by (*2*) and (*4*)

The three axes, radius (*1*), lunate (*2*) and capitate (*3*), are more or less aligned but they hardly ever coincide, the wrist always presenting a certain degree of flexion or extension.

The radiolunate angle (*5*) varies from a dorsiflexion of 25° to a palmar flexion of 10° (average 5° dorsal). The scapholunate angle (*6*) varies from 30° to 60°. Its value is somewhat approximate since determination of the axis of the scaphoid is rather uncertain.

In the case presented, the scapholunate angle is significantly increased: there is dorsiflexion instability of the wrist.

In this second example, note the *scapholunate diastasis* (*1*), although less marked than in the previous case. This configuration can be considered as still being within normal limits, the

35

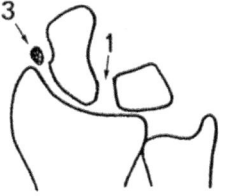 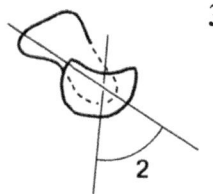

more so that, on a lateral view, the scapholunate angle (*2*) seems normal.

Depending on the movements, and thus also on the positioning during X-raying, the shape of the bones of the first row of the wrist, especially the scaphoid, varies considerably.

An accurate, although still relatively precise study of instability of the wrist can only be performed with a dynamic investigation: frontal view in the neutral position and with ulnar and radial deviation; lateral view in the neutral position and in flexion and in extension; i.e. six radiographs.

The small ossification at the level of the radial styloid process (*3*) is certainly not a traumatic avulsion, even long-standing. It is an accessory ossicle: os radiale externum (cf. No. 13, case 6).

36

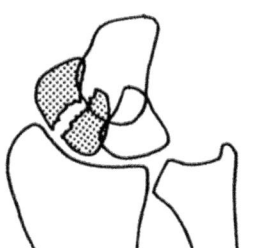 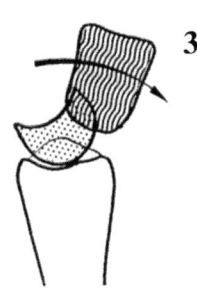

This fracture of the scaphoid is readily recognized. You should have remembered that displacement is uncommon (case 20). The importance of the displacement seen in this case is thus peculiar. Moreover, on the frontal view there is some superimposition of the capitate onto the proximal scaphoid fragment and the lunate.

The lateral view gives evidence of the retrolunate dislocation of the capitate. The diagnosis is thus: *trans-scaphoid retrolunate dislocation* of the wrist.

37

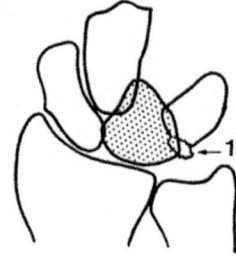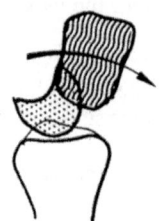

This frontal view again shows the very abnormal overlapping of the lunate on the capitate. On the lateral view the lunate is seen to be tilted volarly and the capitate displaced posteriorly to it. The scaphoid is normal. It is the triquetrum that is fractured; a small fragment of it remains attached to the lunate (*1*), the remaining carpals being displaced backwards. The diagnosis is thus: *trans-triquetral retrolunate displacement of the wrist*.

38

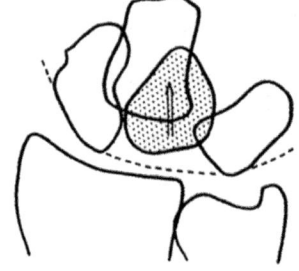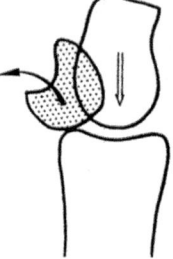

Once again you will recognize on this frontal view the abnormal overlapping of the lunate on the capitate, and on the lateral view the anteriorly tilted lunate.

Unlike in cases 36 and 37, however, the lunate has lost its relationship with the radius. It is enucleated forwards and the rest of the carpal block has regained its place under the radius. This is thus an *anterior dislocation of the lunate*. On the frontal view an important sign is the loss of proximal alignment: scaphoid-lunate-triquetrum. Such a lunate dislocation without associated fracture can easily remain unrecognized, with a diagnosis of "sprain". Now this is very serious because there is a risk of compression of the median nerve in the carpal canal.

Now we can differentiate the two varieties of dislocations of the carpus:

– Anterior dislocation of the lunate: carpal block under the radius and lunate displaced anteriorly
– Retrolunate dislocation of the carpus: lunate under the radius with a fragment of the scaphoid, or, more seldomly, of the triquetrum, and carpal block displaced posteriorly

This diagnosis is readily apparent: it is a transverse fracture of the scaphoid with globally increased density of the two fragments. This increased density corresponds to *post-traumatic-aseptic necrosis,* which occurs only on old fractures, thus on pseudarthrosis. The blood supply in the scaphoid being mainly distal and laterodorsal, only the proximal fragment usually undergoes necrosis. Increased density of the proximal fragment of the scaphoid occurring following a recent fracture may be a sign of necrosis, but can also be encountered at the first stage of a fracture with a favourable evolution. In fact, revascularization may occur from the distal fragment.

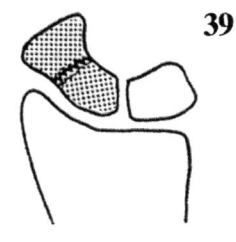

39

Aseptic necrosis of the lunate or Kienböck's disease can be a primary condition, but often occurs following trauma, usually without fracture or dislocation.

The lunate shows increased density and becomes flatter; its proximal margin becomes irregular.

On the distal part of the upper limb osteonecroses have two preferential and almost exclusive locations: the scaphoid and the lunate.

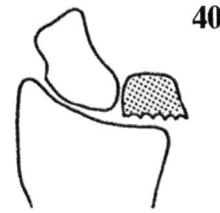

40

Kienböck's disease of the lunate can be:

– Primary (very seldom)
– Following trauma, usually without fracture or dislocation (most often)
– Secondary to a malformation (seldom)

In this case, a short ulna (*1*) provokes disequilibrium in the tensions of the ligaments related to the lunate.

Note that the causal malformation, the ulna minus (*1*), is identical on both sides. On one side only, aseptic necrosis of the lunate has occurred (*2*).

One year later, the lunate is even more flattened and more dense (*3*).

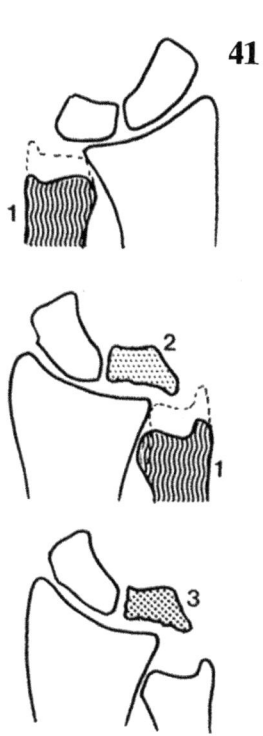

41

42

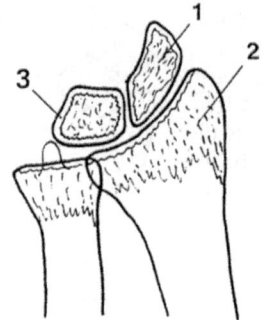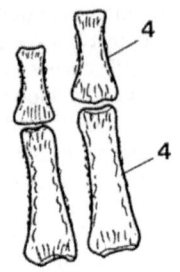

Comparison with the uninvolved side leads to the diagnosis of *algodystrophy* when there are the following radiographic signs:

- Hypertranslucency of the bone, a sign of osteopenia. This is diffuse and homogeneous in the carpal bones (*1*) and epiphyseal and slightly more heterogeneous in the long bones (*2*)
- Subchondral bone resorption visible as a more translucent line (*3*), in particular at the distal end of the radius and the ulna, of certain carpal bones such as the lunate
- Endosteal and subperiosteal cortical bone resorption, which renders the diaphyseal cortices somewhat unsharp (*4*)
- Integrity of the articular interspaces

Radiography is one of the elements in the diagnosis of algodystrophy, the others are pseudoinflammatory clinical syndrome, absence of inflammatory biological data, demineralization visible on X-rays, increased activity on bone scanning, benign evolution and regression without sequels.

There is a history of trauma in half of the cases, for example, inferior radioulnar fracture. One should not make the mistake of considering demineralization as a simple osteoporosis due to immobilization following ablation of the plaster, and rehabilitation would only aggravate the situation. Early diagnosis is difficult. A second site should also be searched for, since shoulder-hand syndromes are classic.

During the regression phase in algodystrophy recalcification occurs with dense and thick trabeculation surrounding bone rarefaction areas, producing a trabeculated appearance with microlacunae distributed somewhat longitudinally on the epiphyses. This is a true stage of sequellar atrophy or of healing of the algodystrophy. The cortical bone still shows reduced thickness, and compared with the uninvolved side the carpus is more translucent. This appearance can persist throughout life; but sometimes the radiological signs disappear after a few years.

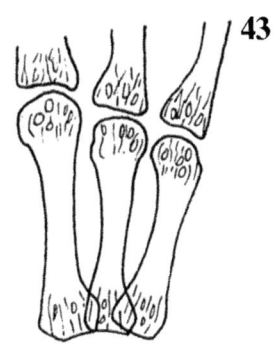

43

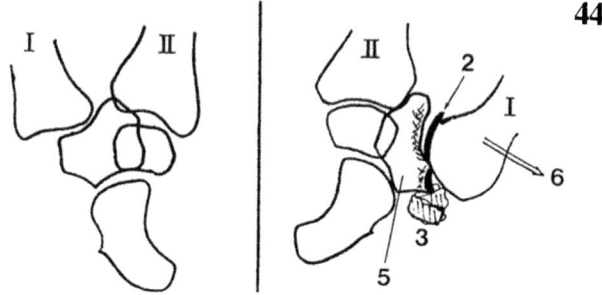

44

Trapezometacarpal arthrosis of the thumb is the most frequent site of degeneration rheumatic disease on the hand. The frontal view of the hand is the view usually available but it gives an oblique view of the trapezometacarpal joint. For a more accurate study, strict lateral and frontal views according to Kapandji are necessary. Nevertheless, one must also be able to make the diagnosis of trapezometacarpal arthrosis or rhizarthrosis from a frontal view. For this purpose we search for the following radiological signs:

- Narrowing of the articular interspace (*1*)
- Subchondral densification of the articular surfaces (*2*)
- More or less hypertrophic osteophytosis on the radial aspect of the trapezium and around the metacarpal base (*3*)
- Lacunae in the trapezium and metacarpal (*4*)
- Deformation of the trapezium (*5*)
- Outward subluxation of the metacarpal with progressive spreading of the base of the first and second metacarpals (*6*)

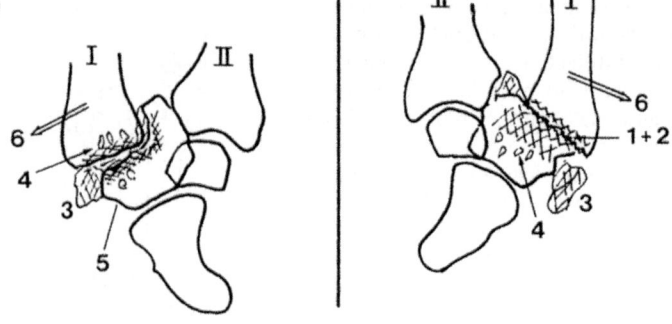

Not all the radiological signs of trapezometacarpal arthrosis of the thumb are present in case 44. This next bilateral case is much more advanced and shows the entire radiological semiology.

In addition, we note again the isolated character of these degenerative changes in the wrist.

With regard to the spreading of the base of the first and second metacarpals, caution is advised. Indeed, slight spreading can be considered as a normal variant related to a somewhat accentuated development of the tubercle of the trapezium. In the relatively advanced cases 44 and 45 subluxation is, however, indisputable.

Digital arthrosis involves mainly the distal interphalangeal, more rarely the proximal interphalangeal, and, exceptionally, the metacarpophalangeal joints. Digital involvement begins, and later predominates, usually on the index. The radiological changes are the same in all digital arthrosic localizations:

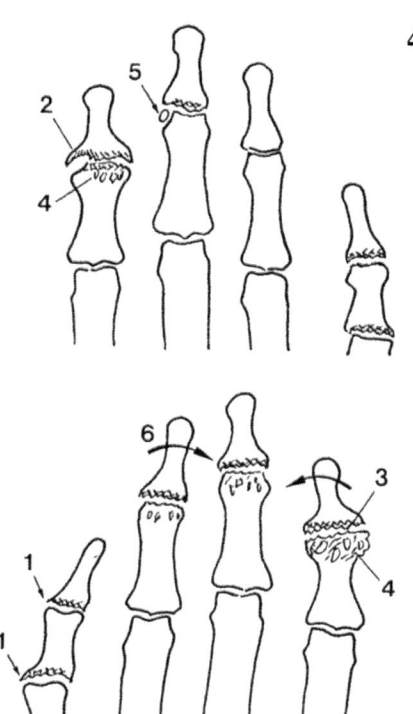

- Osteophyte formation: first small pointed spurs (*1*), then hypertrophic formations (*2*), inserted on the head of the phalanx and mainly on the base of the adjacent phalanx. These osteophytes form mainly on the lateral edges and on the dorsal aspect. They correspond to Heberden nodes in the distal interphalangeal joints and to Bouchard nodes in the proximal interphalangeal joints. Osteophytes are the dominant radiological feature
- Narrowing of the joint space (*3*)
- Subchondral erosion with lacunae and increased density areas (*4*)
- Ossification of the joint capsule (*5*)
- Deformation of the joints, usually deviation towards the middle finger (*6*) and even true subluxations.

Digital arthroses are often rather well tolerated in spite of the very marked deformations. On the contrary, trapezometacarpal arthrosis of the thumb often causes severe functional disturbances.

47

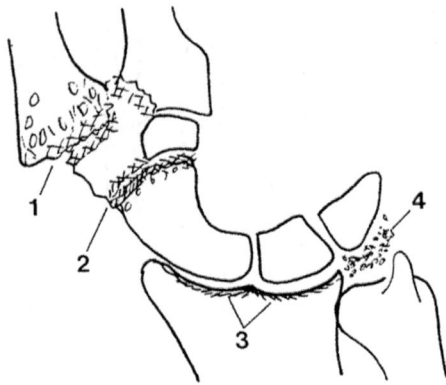

Multiple radiological anomalies are visible on this wrist:

- You will have of course recognized advanced trapezometacarpal arthrosis (*1*)
- *Scaphotrapezial arthropathy* (*2*) with narrowed joint space and subchondral osteosclerosis, a much more unusual sign for "arthrosis"
- Narrowing of the radiocarpal joint (*3*) is often difficult to appreciate because the vertical beam does not permit its correct visualization. With the hand flat, palm down, a 30° ascendant beam would be necessary to clear the radial glenoid cavity from the scaphoid and lunate. Nevertheless, we see on this radiograph a double imprint of the scaphoid and lunate, suggesting at least a narrowing of the radiocarpal joint
- In the space between the distal end of the ulna and the triquetrum note the thin calcifications corresponding to the *triangular cartilage of the carpus* (*4*)

Calcifications of the triangular cartilage of the carpus and presence of scaphotrapezial arthropathy lead to the conclusion of *articular chondrocalcinosis.*

48

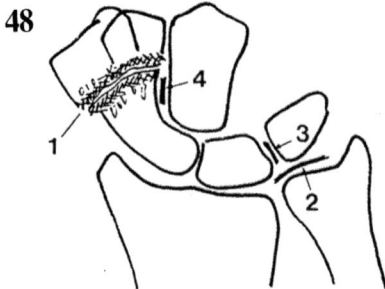

Articular chondrocalcinosis is a metabolic rheumatic disease comprising deposits of dihydrate pyrophosphates in the articular cartilage and fibrocartilages, the synovia and the joint capsule, and chronic arthropathies resembling, from the radiological point of view, arthrosis.

Since there is no concomitant arthrosis, the present case is much more characteristic. Note:

- The scaphotrapezial and trapezoid arthropathy (*1*), which is very typical with the narrowed joint space, the subchondral bone sclerosis and erosion over the head of scaphoid
- Calcification of the triangular cartilage of the carpus (fibrocartilage) (*2*)
- Intercarpal calcifications between the lunate and the triquetrum (*3*) and between the scaphoid and the capitate (*4*) (articular cartilages)

In articular chondrocalcinosis the most characteristic abnormality is the *calcification of the triangular cartilage* of the carpus.

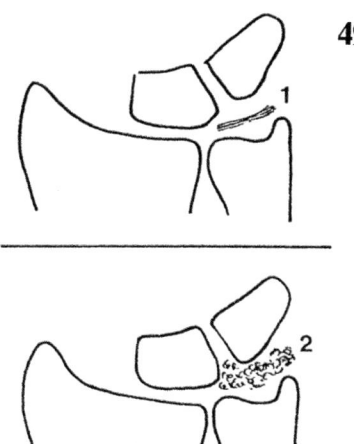

49

It is seen either as a roughly linear stratified opacity (*1*) or as a more or less voluminous granulous accumulation (*2*) which may extend beyond the joint space (case 50).

One must now search for the two other characteristic locations:

– Meniscocalcinosis and calcinosis of the articular cartilage in the knees
– Calcification of the fibrocartilage in the symphysis pubis characterized by a linear calcification running down the centre of the symphysis

Simultaneous involvement of the three main sites makes the diagnosis.

Unlike in the previous case, we find here all the radiological signs of chondrocalcinosis:

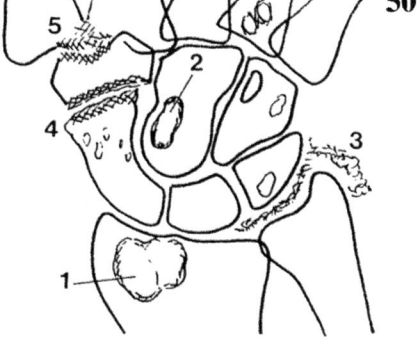

50

– Multiple erosions, some of them voluminous, in the radial epiphysis (*1*) and the capitate (*2*); other smaller ones in the scaphoid, the triquetrum, the hamate and the base of the fourth metacarpal
– Very extensive calcification of the triangular cartilage (*3*)
– Finally, scaphoidotrapezial (*4*) and trapezometacarpal (*5*) arthropathies, still slightly destructive.

Because of the concomitance of the other signs of chondrocalcinosis, the trapezometacarpal involvement must be considered in this case as belonging to the same aetiological group.

51

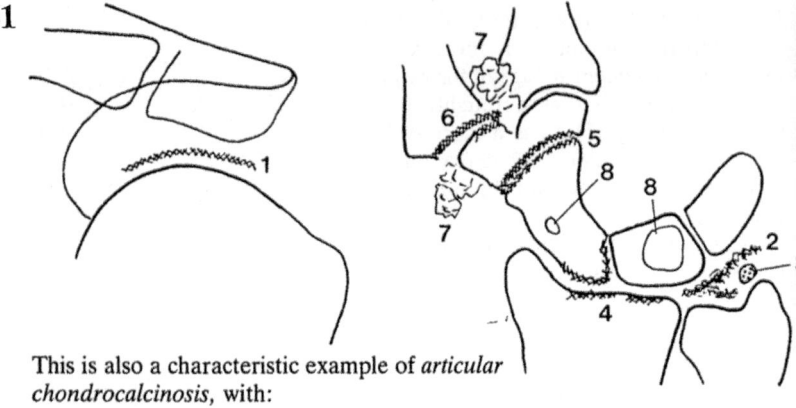

This is also a characteristic example of *articular chondrocalcinosis,* with:

– Calcification of the articular cartilage of the humeral head (*1*)
– Calcification of the triangular cartilage of the carpus (*2*) close to an accessory ossicle we know well: the os triangulare (*3*)
– Radiocarpal (*4*) scaphotrapezial and trapezoid (*5*) and trapezometacarpal (*6*) arthropathies
– Hypertrophic osteophytosis on the radial edge of the trapezium and around the metacarpal base (*7*), a configuration we have already seen in arthrosis (case 44)
– Micro- and macroerosions (*8*)

52

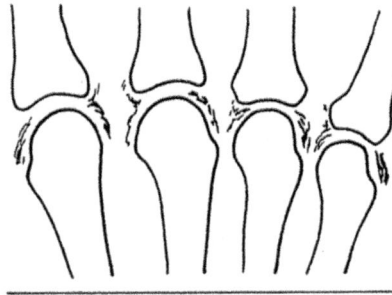

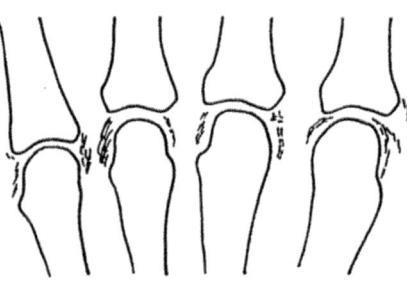

Besides the carpus, articular chondrocalcinosis also involves, although less commonly (20%), *the metacarpophalangeal joints.* Involvement is usually bilateral from the second to the fifth finger. It almost always accompanies other localizations, in particular the triangular cartilage of the carpus.

The calcifications here are mainly lateral, involving the *capsulosynovial membrane,* partly outlining the capsular contour.

These calcifications are just as frequent on the radial as on the ulnar side of each joint. Metacarpophalangeal involvements are very characteristic and should never be mistaken for manifestations of rheumatoid arthritis.

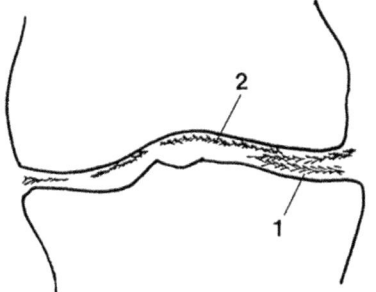 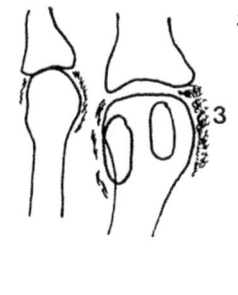

In this patient the radiological anomalies are almost the same on both sides and very characteristic of *articular chondrocalcinosis:*

– On the metacarpophalangeal joints: calcified synovium and capsules with intact joint spaces and articular surfaces
– On the knees: calcifications of the meniscus (*1*) and of the articular cartilage (*2*). Meniscocalcinosis occurs frequently after the age of 60 years, and is thus, by itself, insufficient to affirm the diagnosis of chondrocalcinosis
– On the metatarsophalangeal joints: tendinoligamentous and capsulosynovial periarticular calcifications (*3*) also with intact joint spaces and articular surfaces. Involvement of the feet is much rarer than that of the hands

Let us point out here that there is no parallel between the clinical and the radiological signs: pain may exist when the joints are radiologically normal, and vice versa.

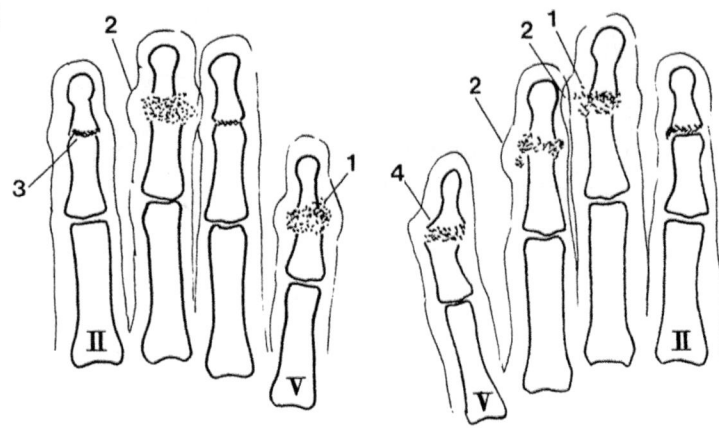

You should have noted the following radiological changes:

- Multiple small periarticular calcifications, on most of the distal interphalangeal joints (*1*), whereas the proximal and the metacarpophalangeal joints are normal. These calcifications are numerous, very dense, homogeneous, granulous or linear
- Swelling of the soft parts at the level of the involved joints (*2*)
- Erosions over several small joints (*3*), some of them showing deformity and disalignment (*4*)

In the presence of erosive arthropathies and circumscribed calcinoses, different diagnostic possibilities must be discussed:

1. *Rheumatoid arthritis with hydroxyapatite* or *multiple tendon calcifications disease*. This is a metabolic disorder belonging to the group of the microcrystalline arthritis for the same reason as articular chondrocalcinosis and gout. Often asymptomatic or characterized by trivial algiae, this affection predominates, in order of decreasing frequency, in the shoulder, the hip and the hand. Hydroxyapatite crystals are deposited in the periarticular structures: articular capsule, ligaments and tendons. On the hands the sites affected are usually the distal interphalangeal joints and the carpus at the level of the radial and ulnar styloid processes. Calcifications are, however, usually less numerous than in the case presented here, and the joint is only involved in long-standing cases.

2. *Destructive arthrosis.* The periarticular calcifications here are much denser than in arthrosic ossifications, and there are no osteophytes.

3. *Sclerodermia.* There are no signs of atrophy of the extremities (fingertips, tufts of the distal phalanges). Moreover, arthropathies are far less numerous in scleroderma.

4. *Hyperparathyroidism.* Here, the bone structures are normal. Moreover, in hyperparathyroidism calcifications are more voluminous.

For this case the definitive diagnosis remains disputable between an unusual variant of arthrosis and an uncommon form of hydroxyapatitic rheumatoid arthritis.

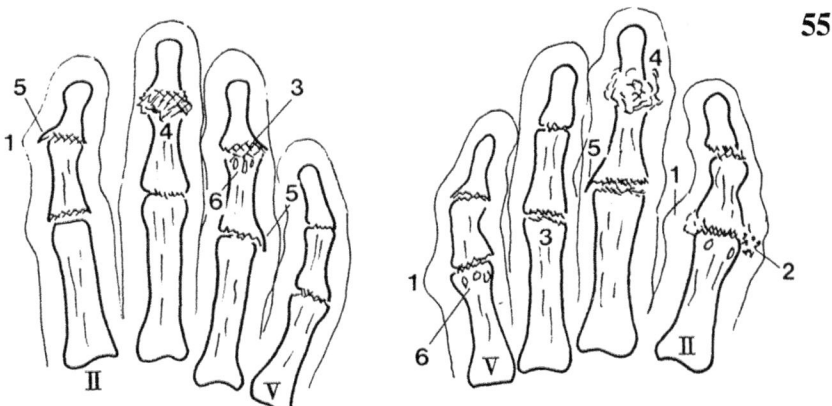

All the interdigital joints are involved in this case, although to different degrees. The following features are noted:

- Thickened soft parts (*1*) and in some places thin calcifications corresponding to tophic masses (*2*)
- Narrowed joint spaces (*3*)
- Articular destructions (*4*)
- Osteophytes (*5*)
- Defects in the bone extremities (*6*)
- Overall osteopororis with thinning of the cortical bone, bone hypertranslucency and slightly dense appearance of the longitudinal bone trabeculations

This is certainly not a case of rheumatoid arthritis, since the metacarpophalangeal joints are spared. Neither is it an arthrosis; when compared with case 46, the lesions here are more destructive and the thickening of the soft parts adjacent to the joints does not correspond to subjacent hypertrophic osteophytes. The diagnosis of *chronic gout* is thus obvious.

Although the tophi have a radiological opacity similar to that of the soft tissues, they are responsible for the bumpy swellings randomly distributed over several fingers. Narrowing and destruction of joints result respectively from destruction of the cartilage due to deposition of urate crystals, and from subchondral defects in the bone extremities. Peripheral and usually small osteophytes are the sign of the osteocartilaginous reaction.

Uratic arthropathies involve mainly the distal part of the foot, the carpus and the fingers, the ankle, the knee and the elbow.

56

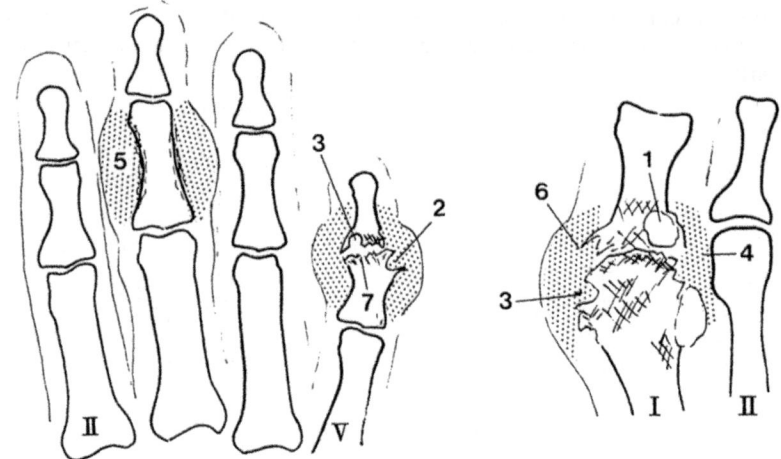

Chronic uratic arthropathy here is much more characteristic with its selective localization to the metatarsophalangeal joint of the first toe and its ubiquitous distribution on the hand. In this case, the radiological semiology is complete:

– Central defects expanding the bone (*1*) and lateral epiphyseal (*2*) and subchondral, more or less confluent defects eroding the articular surface (*3*)
– Tophi in the soft parts adjacent to the joints (*4*) or distant from them with periosteal reaction (*5*)
– Osteophytes (*6*)
– Erosion and destruction of joints (*7*)

After several years of treatment aimed at decreasing the amount of uric acid, the initial roentgen manifestations of uratic arthropathy can change progressively: decreased size of the tophi, diminution or disappearance of defects and indentations, and restitution of an almost normal joint space.

57

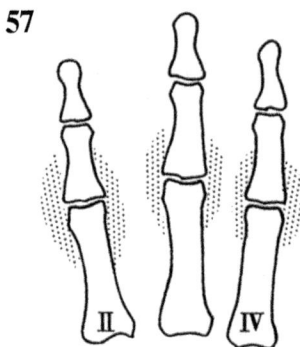

If you have come to the conclusion that this is a normal image, you are wrong. In fact you should have taken into account the increased thickness and opacity of the soft parts adjacent to the proximal interphalangeal joints.

This is a case of *rheumatoid arthritis* in its onset phase with *rheumatoid synovitis*. The joint spaces are still normal.

The second early sign is the increased radiolucency of the epiphyses in the metacarpophalangeal and proximal interphalangeal joints due to osteoporosis related to inactivity and local hyperemia which accompany synovial inflammation.

The first localized bone signs appearing in *rheumatoid arthritis* on the metacarpophalangeal joints are the following:

- Rounded or ovalar defects (*1*) of less than 5 mm, with sharp or unsharp margins, sometimes with a dense sclerotic border. They are located in the subchondral bone, mainly in the metacarpal heads or in the carpal bones
- Erosions, on the lateral aspect and mainly on the radial side, at the site of the capsulosynovial insertion, on the metacarpal head (*2*) as well as on the base of the phalanx (*3*), on the junction of the subchondral bone lamina and on the cortical bone
- Narrowing of the joint spaces (*4*), a sign of cartilage destruction. This sign is of major importance for the diagnosis and prognosis insofar as changes in the cartilage are irreversible. It is, however, difficult to affirm the presence of joint narrowing when this is moderate: the least flexion may be responsible for a false narrowing image

On the most severely involved joint (second metacarpophalangeal) the adjacent soft parts are markedly thickened (*5*). Epiphyseal osteoporosis remains moderate.

59

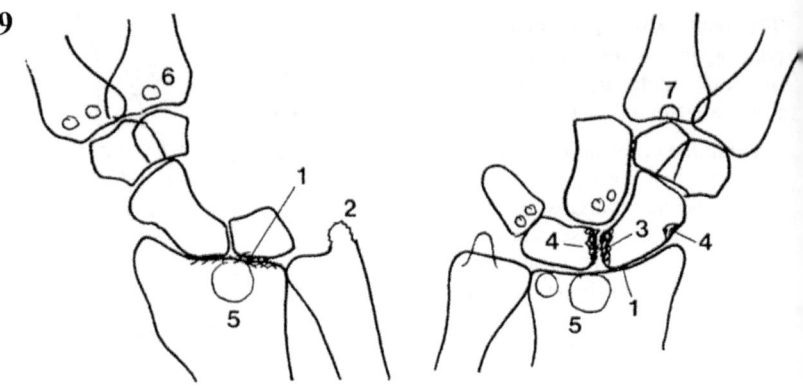

The carpus, also, becomes affected early in *rheumatoid arthritis:*

– Demineralization of the carpal bones, radial and ulnar epiphyses, and metacarpal bases
– Narrowing of the radiocarpal (*1*) and intracarpal joints, the latter being more difficult to visualize and depending on the positioning of the hand
– The earliest occurring bone erosions are most often seen on the radial styloid process (*2*) and the proximal border of the scaphoid (*4*) but any other site can be affected
– Ubiquitously distributed defects. They are often of rather large size in the radial epiphysis (*5*). They can also be located in the spongiosa (*6*) or at the level of the subchondral lamina (*7*). These defects are not really specific of rheumatoid arthritis. Trivial dystrophic defects can often be seen in the carpal bones, mainly in the scaphoid and capitate, and their frequency increases with age.

The dominant feature in this radiographic image is the presence of numerous bilateral defects. Most of them are distributed over the carpal bones and the metacarpal heads. They are rounded or oval shaped, central or peripheral, with or without a sclerotic margin and of unequal size, some over 5 mm.

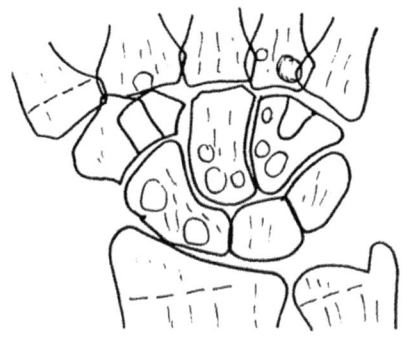

The second abnormality is the dense trabeculated appearance of the spongious bone, due to a certain degree of remineralization. The bone contours are unaffected. There are neither erosions nor joint narrowings.

Some traces of the growth cartilage persist on the epiphyses of the first metacarpal, the radius and the ulna. This case concerns a young adult who had had *juvenile rheumatoid arthritis* for several years.

Whatever the variety of juvenile rheumatoid arthritis, i.e. systemic form of Still's disease, mono or oligoarthritis, or progressive polyarticular form, the roentgen changes are rather unvarying and

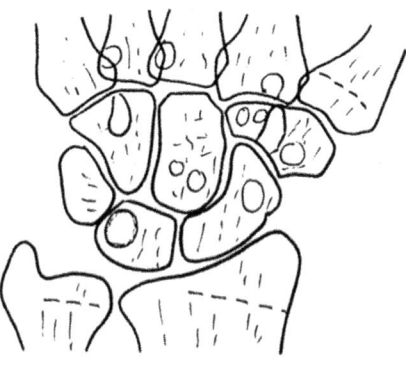

very similar to those seen in adults. There are moreover the disturbances due to bone growth. We may thus encounter: osteoporosis (constant, frequent, diffuse), periosteal appositions on the metacarpal diaphyses fused with the cortex, narrowed joint spaces, erosions and defects (occurring later); bone maturation is often retarded but may sometimes be accelerated causing premature closure of the metacarpal epiphyses with subsequent brachymetacarpia. Development of the disease can stop at any stage without this ensuring definite stabilization. There is then stabilization in the radiographic changes, partial regression of osteoporosis and reappearance of some regularity in the density and contours of the carpal bones. This is what we see in case 60.

Note moreover that juvenile rheumatoid arthritis predominates over the hands, but also involves, in decreasing order of frequency, the cervical spine, the temporomandibular joint, the hips and the sacroiliac joints.

61

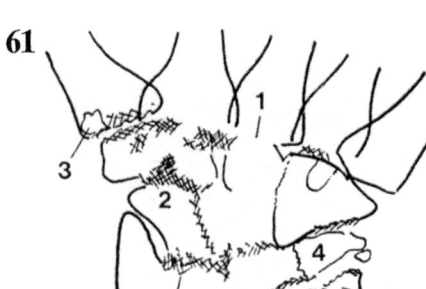

In *advanced rheumatoid arthritis,* one can see a stage with *carpal fusion:*

– Disappearance of the joint spaces (*1*)
– Ragged, notched and dense appearance of the subchondral bone (*2*)
– Defects (*3*)
– Bone deformations and flattening (*4*)

The radiographic image is thus clearly different from that of arthrosis, in particular on the metacarpophalangeal joint of the thumb, and from arthropathies in articular chondrocalcinosis.

62
63

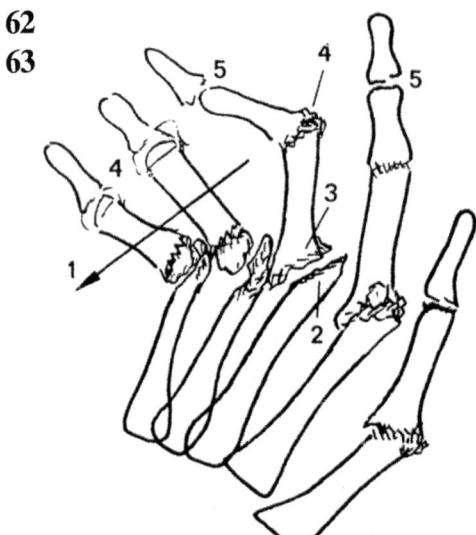

In *long-standing* and advanced forms of *rheumatoid arthritis* there exist, besides carpal fusion, severely deforming arthropathies of the fingers:

– Subluxation and, later, luxation of the proximal phalanges (*1*) deviated towards the ulna and in flexion
– Erosion of the metacarpal heads which have become pointed (*2*)
– Cupuliform appearance of the phalangeal base (*3*)
– Deformation of the proximal interphalangeal joints with hyperextension (*4*)
– Unaffected distal interphalangeal joints (*5*)

Destruction is in this case even more advanced with total disappearance of the carpal bones and real atrophic osteolysis of all the epiphyseal extremities and, paradoxically, unaffected distal interphalangeal joints.

The differential diagnosis should be discussed with regard to:
– Lupus: involvements are more distal, quite as destructive but less often affect the carpus
– Syringomyelia: less-deforming, more destructive, mainly distal atrophy of the phalanges; also affects the elbow
– Ulcero-mutilating acropathy: occurs more commonly on the foot.

Radiographs *A* and *B* represent the same hand X-rayed at an interval of 8 months.

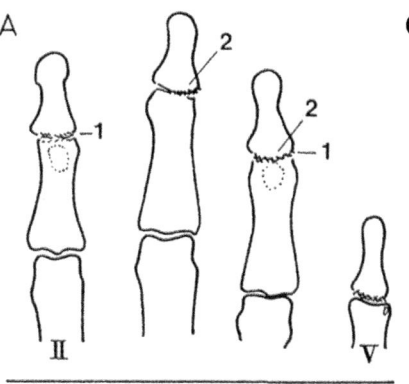

On radiograph *A* you note:
- The exclusive involvement of the distal interphalangeal joints
- Narrowing of the joint spaces due to degeneration of the articular cartilages (*1*)
- Irregularity and densification of the subchondral bone (*2*)
- The epiphyses and phalangeal bases are not osteoporotic

Eight months later radiograph *B* shows significant aggravation, with:

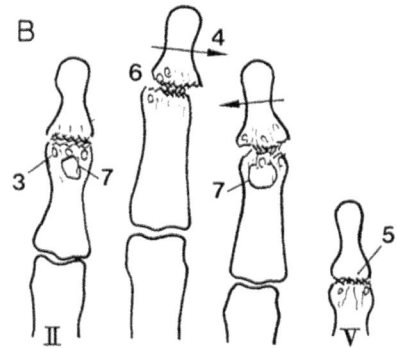

- Appearance of subchondral microlacunae (*3*)
- Deviation of some distal phalanges (*4*)
- Aggravation of the joint narrowing (*5*) and of the erosions, mainly around the distal interphalangeal space on the third finger (*6*)
- Two large defects (*7*) the presence of which had only been tentatively guessed on the initial radiograph

The exclusive involvement of the distal interphalangeal joints rules out rheumatoid arthritis. The radiosemiology is, however, the same. This is a *psoriatic arthropathy*.

Psoriatic rheumatism can be of two varieties: an evolutive chronic polyarticular process, with peripheral changes predominantly on the hands and feet, but with characteristic differences, and, on the other hand, rheumatic pelvispondylitis, thus affecting the axial skeleton in isolation or in association with arthritides of the limbs.

There are two possibilities:
- Cutaneous psoriasis is present: this is the commonest case. The diagnosis is based on the following triad "inflammatory articular changes + cutaneous psoriasis + negative rheumatoid serology"
- There is no history of cutaneous psoriasis: the diagnosis is then based on seronegative polyarthritis in peripheral involvements and rheumatic pelvispondylitis in the axial involvements.

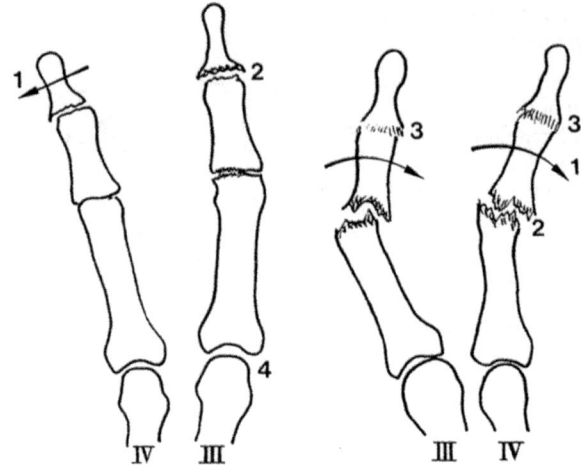

Psoriatic arthropathy is incorrectly believed to involve only the distal interphalangeal joints. During the evolution, which is often more rapid than with rheumatoid arthritis, the same radiological changes appear. It is, however, true that in rheumatoid arthritis the distal interphalangeal joints remain uninvolved, whereas in psoriatic arthritis the metacarpophalangeal joints are spared.

Note in this case:
- Ulnar subluxation (*1*)
- Erosive arthritis (*2*)
- Articular ankyloses (*3*)
- Intact metacarpophalangeal joints (*4*)

In psoriatic arthropathy on the hands, one can also find bony proliferations such as osteophytes and periostal proliferations around the diaphyses and the capsulotendinous insertion areas.

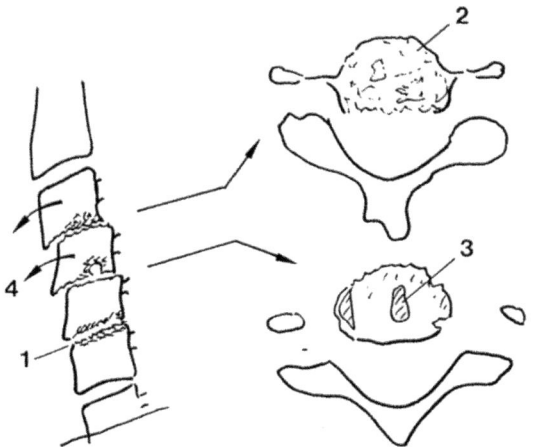

When you compare these hands and those of case 62 you will see the analogies and the differences which allow diagnosis respectively of rheumatoid arthritis (case 62) and psoriatic arthropathy (case 66):

- Almost similar carpal fusion
- More or less identical destructive arthropathies but differently located: metacarpophalangeal and proximal interphalangeal in rheumatoid arthritis, proximal and distal interphalangeal in psoriatic arthropathy
- Subluxations towards the ulna and luxations of the fingers but at different levels, depending on the joints involved

In this same patient, cervical spine radiographs showed:
- Spondylodiscitis from C3 to C6 with narrowed intervertebral spaces (*1*), unsharp erosion of the vertebral plates (*2*) and subchondral defects (*3*). These spondylodiscites progressively develop into a vertebral block
- Anterior subluxation of C3 and C4 (*4*)
- Absence of syndesmophytes. In fact, these are characteristic of ankylosing spondylarthritis. In psoriatic arthropathy, depending on whether the affection is closer to rheumatoid arthritis or to ankylosing spondylarthritis, the cervical involvement takes on the appearance of one or the other of these affections. Since in case 66 the lesions on the hands are mainly peripheral, the rheumatoid arthritis type form is present, which *never* shows syndesmophytes.

67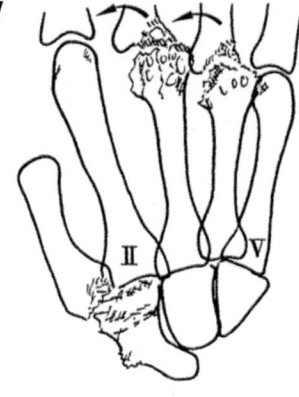

On both hands there is clear evidence of trapezometacarpal arthropathy of the thumb resembling trivial degenerative arthrosis. However, marked involvement, on one hand, of the metacarpophalangeal joints of the third and fourth fingers must lead to a diagnosis of *polyarthritis*.

There are clear discrepancies in this case with regard to rheumatoid arthritis. The lesion at the base of the thumb could be consistent with ancient arthrosis. The metacarpophalangeal joints are not all affected and the symmetrical right-left involvement, common in rheumatoid arthritis, does not exist here. Moreover, the subluxation of the two affected fingers is towards the radius. Also the rheumatoid serology was negative. The case presented is thus *seronegative polyarthritis*.

68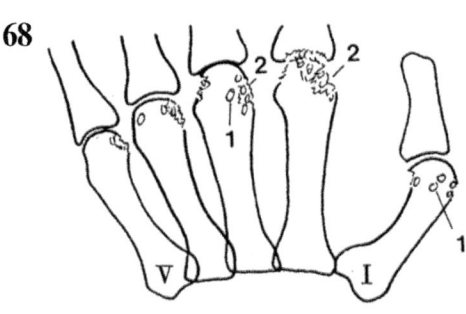

You will have certainly noted a number of similarities with case 67:

– Multiple microdefects (*1*) in the metacarpal heads, especially in the lateral part on the radial side
– Lateral erosions about the synovial recesses of the metacarpal heads (*2*)

The radiological changes are about similar on both sides and involve all the metacarpophalangeal joints.

This is thus a case of polyarthritis resembling rheumatoid arthritis. In fact, we see here the presence of chronic polyarthritis in *systemic lupus erythematosus*.

It must be kept in mind that acute, subacute or chronic articular manifestations are present in 90% of cases and that they are the revealing factor in one out of two cases. Chronic polyarthritis can affect only the synovia and can cause neither deformations nor roentgen changes. It can also simulate rheumatoid arthritis with involvement of the metacarpophalangeal and proximal interphalangeal joints. There are divergent opinions concerning the severity of the affection, but lupic arthritis can be said to cause more deformities and more destruction than trivial rheumatoid arthritis.

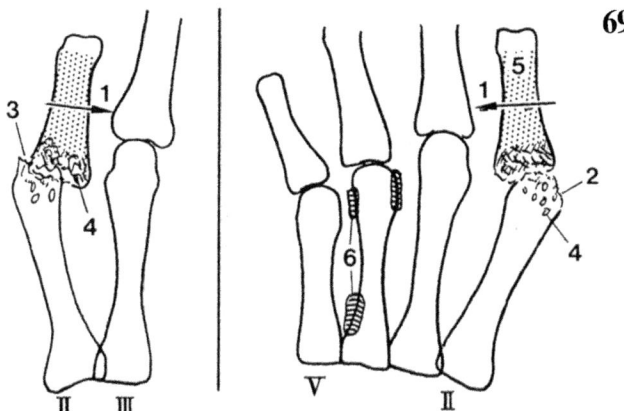

The association of an oligoarthritis with multiple calcifications about the soft parts evokes a *collagen disease*.

The arthritides affect here solely the second metacarpophalangeal joint on each side, and in an almost similar way:

- Luxation towards the ulna and flexion of the proximal phalanx (*1*)
- Erosion of the lateral edges of the metacarpal head over the lateral synovial recesses (*2*)
- Destruction of the subchondral bone (*3*)
- Defects in the metacarpal head and phalangeal base (*4*)
- Sclerosing remodeling of the bone structure in the entire proximal phalanx (*5*), very marked by comparison with the homologous phalanx of the third finger

There are few *calcifications* in the soft parts of the hand (*6*) and many more in the other areas, as for instance the concretions seen in the inguinal, crural region.

This is a case of *dermatomyositis*. Called polymyositis when there are no cutaneous lesions and dermomyositis when the skin changes are dominant, this collagenosis comprises, in one-third of cases, articular manifestations, either mere polyarthralgiae or true polyarthritis, mainly around the extremities. A stage of pure synovitis, without X-ray changes, is followed by a phase with destructive and mutilating arthropathy.

70 This real calcinosis of the soft parts of both hands and one forearm indicates a diagnosis of *Thibierge-Weissenbach syndrome,* also described as the *CRST syndrome,* i.e. subcutaneous calcinosis – Raynaud – sclerodactyly – telangiectasia. It is thus a clinical form of *scleroderma.*

The Thibierge-Weissenbach syndrome is present in about 10%–12% of scleroderma, and often rather early (some years) in the evolution of the disease. Raynaud syndrome and telangiectasia can occur before signs of scleroderma exist.

Calcinosis is the most characteristic sign. On the hands it develops selectively from the metacarpophalangeal joints to the fingertips. Involvement of elbows and forearms is less frequent, of hips and toes still more uncommon. On the fingers the site is subcutaneous and more seldom musculoaponeurotic. Usually the articular structures themselves are unaffected (capsule, ligaments, synovia). Intra-articular calcium deposits have been described as an uncommon occurrence, associated with articular erosion, leading rapidly to mutilating arthropathy. The calcifications are of variable size; some of them may reach 10–15 mm, especially over the elbow. They have a tendency to form clusters, but can also remain scattered. These deposits consist of calcium phosphate and carbonate, thus of hydroxyapatite.

The distal phalanges of the fingers also show sclerodactyly, but in this case we were concerned mainly with the calcinosis. Sclerodactyly is better displayed in the following case (71).

71

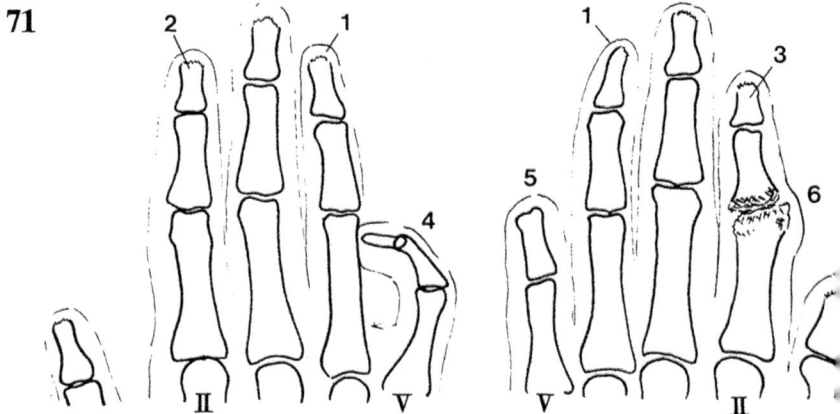

This case of *scleroderma* has no calcifications of the soft parts. There are, however, several characteristic abnormalities:

– Atrophy of the fingertips (*1*)
– Erosion and progressive resorption of the tufts of the distal phalanges (*2*). Destruction will lead to the progressive disappearance of the phalanx in the proximal direction (*3*)

156

- Retractile atrophy of the skin, progressively impeding the joint mobility. Some fingers are fixed in the flexed position (4) and become thin and ulcerated; amputations may become necessary (5)
- More uncommon deforming arthropathy (6). About one-third of patients with scleroderma also have chronic oligo- or polyarthritides, characterized by moderate or absence of pain and inflammatory changes, and by the absence of rheumatoid nodosities.

In scleroderma the dominant feature about the hands is the *sclerodactylia*. Arthritides and calcinosis in the soft parts are much rarer.

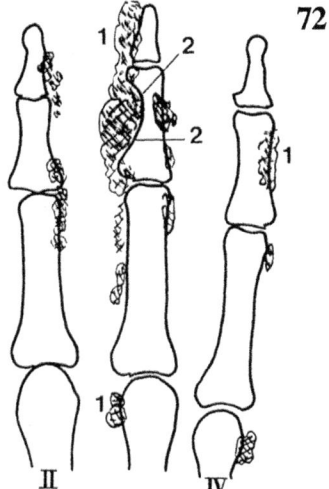

72

This important calcinosis in the soft parts of the elbow and fingers is not caused by a collagen disease. In fact, besides the major collagen diseases (scleroderma, polymyositis), other different pathological conditions comprise calcium deposits in the soft parts over the fingers: primary hypercalcaemia, hyperparathyroidism, chronic renal insufficiency and, more particularly, pseudogout in haemodyalized patients.

The case presented here is in fact *calcic pseudogout in a patient with haemodyalysis*. The signs of *hyperparathyroidism secondary to chronic renal insufficiency* are dominated by the importance of the so-called metastatic calcifications of the soft parts (1), clinically mimicking uratic arthropathy tophi, although they are much denser.

Note also on the middle phalanx of the third finger resorption of the radial aspect (2) adjacent to voluminous calcium deposits.

73

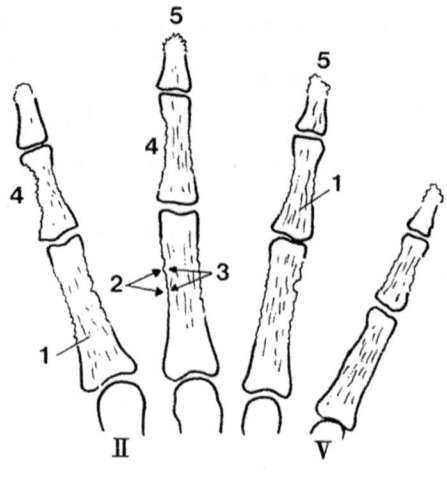

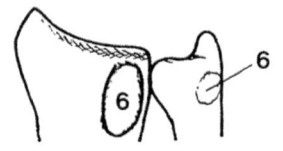

Primary hyperparathyroidism causes very characteristic changes on the hands:

- Diffuse osteoporosis with globally decreased bone density
- Dense and irregular longitudinal bone trabeculations in the medulla (*1*) providing, in spite of the presence of osteoporosis, the appearance of densifying osteoporosis
- Subperiosteal (*2*) and endosteal (*3*) resorption, causing thinning of the cortical margin and widening of the medullary cavities, mainly over the proximal phalanges. There is more marked subperiosteal resorption on the middle phalanges, especially on the radial aspect of the second and third fingers (*4*)
- Erosion and progressive resorption of the tuft of the distal phalanges (*5*) as in scleroderma but without atrophy of the fingertips
- Rounded or oval-shaped lucent defects, with or without sclerotic margin, mainly over the radial and ulnar epiphyses (*6*). These defects are also very characteristic in the skull vault where they are often quite numerous and must not be mistaken for Paget's disease or multiple myeloma

In the presence of such data of primary hyperparathyroidism, radiological investigations should also be performed to search for urinary calculi and for nephrocalcinosis. Note also that the bony signs are present in only about 50% of the cases with primary hyperparathyroidism. After exeresis of the parathyroid lesion, remineralization of the skeleton is quite rapid. Case 73 is quite a convincing example when you compare the skull vault before (*A*) and 2 months after (*B*) surgical removal of the adenoma.

You will now be able to recognize the signs of *primary hyperparathyroidism,* and the present case is just as characteristic as the previous:

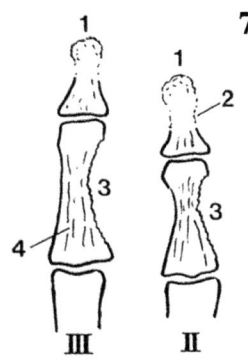

– Distal phalanges tuft erosion (*1*)
– Subperiosteal and endosteal resorption about the diaphyses producing the disappearance of a great part of the bone of the distal phalanges (*2*)
– Marked subperiosteal resorption over the radial aspect of the middle phalanx of the second and third fingers (*3*)
– Dense and coarse bone trabeculations in the spongiosa (*4*), producing the appearance of diffuse osteosclerosis

The vertebral involvement is just as typical: increased translucency due to demineralization (increased osteoclast activity), unsharp appearance of the remaining bone structure, collapse of the vertebral bodies and very closely mimicking osteomalacia.

This case is clearly different from the two previous ones. There is, indeed, no alteration of the bone contours, in particular over the tuft of the distal phalanges, and around the diaphyses of the other phalanges. There is only one radiological sign: *the increased translucency of the bone.* It is global and massive, with rarefaction of the bone trabeculations in the spongiosa and thinning of the cortical bone. Note that the growth cartilage is still visible, and that one of the sesamoids of the thumb, at least, is present. The bone age is thus approximately 12–14 years.

Such a global increased translucency of the bone may correspond to various aetiologies: osteoporosis due to corticoids, deficiency osteomalacia, haemopathy, etc. Here the diagnosis was *enterogenous osteopathy caused by a malabsorption syndrome.* The radiological findings on the hands are thus unspecific.

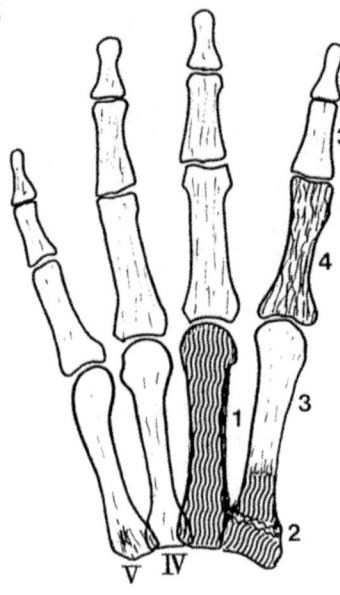

The radiological changes seen on the hands of this elderly female patient are much more subtle: You should have noted:

- Almost complete sclerosis of the third metacarpal; only the head is spared, with a slight thickening around the diaphyses (*1*)
- Fracture on the proximal part of the diaphysis of the second metacarpal (*2*) with sclerosis of the adjacent areas. As this site is definitely unusual, the fracture must be considered pathological
- Osteoporosis of the entire digital axis below the fracture (*3*)
- Coarse and sclerotic trabecular remodelling in the entire proximal phalanx of the second finger (*4*)

Modifications *1–4* are characteristic of Paget's disease although involvement of the hand (metacarpal, proximal phalangeal) is exceptional. The sclerosis of the third metacarpal must, however, lead to this diagnosis although fracture of the second metacarpal is more difficult to explain, since there are no other remodelling signs in this bone. The author concluded that it was fatigue fracture.

Without difficulty, you will note here:

- Coarse and irregular trabeculation pattern in the spongy bone of metacarpals and phalanges
- Diffusedly increased density of the carpal bones
- Symmetrical and similar involvement of both hands
- Condensing osteitis of the ulna (*1*) and radius (*2*), and ossification of the upper and middle part of the interosseous membrane (*3*)
- Condensing osteitis of the cervical vertebrae

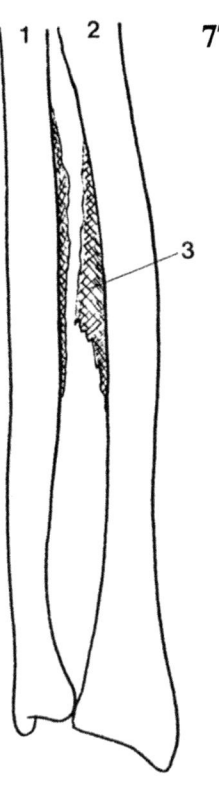

There is thus evidence of a general condensing affection of the whole skeleton or condensing osteosis. By condensing osteosis is meant a transformation of the bone due to increased formation or to excessive mineralization, or also by abnormal medullary sclerosis, but of the non-inflammatory, non-infectious, non-malignant cytoproliferative type. Among the generalized forms, some condensing osteoses are congenital and have their own radiological characteristics, enabling their precise diagnosis to be made; for example, Albers-Schoenberg osteopetrosis, pyknodysostosis and hyperostotic osteopathy of Camurati-Engelmann. Others are acquired affections, secondary to diverse causes: skeletal fluorosis, hyperparathyroidism and myelosclerosis.

Our patient is suffering from hydrotelluric *fluorosis*, caused by a high fluoride level in the drinking water. This intoxication is especially seen in some regions of northern Africa and in India. The disease is frequently latent and sometimes revealed by osteoarticular pain. There is a general symmetrical involvement of the skeleton, with axial predominance (spine, pelvis). A very typical sign is the ossification of the radioulnar interosseous membrane.

78

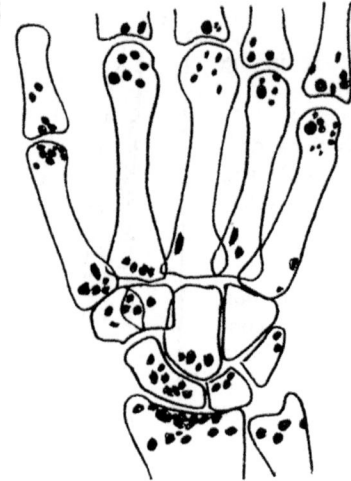

The multiple small bone condensations, rounded or oval shaped, distributed more or less symmetrically over both hands, and seen also in one shoulder, have enabled the diagnosis of *osteopoikilosis* to be made. This is in fact the only possibility which can be discussed from the radiological point of view.

This "disease" is rather a radiological curiosity. It is classified with osteochondrodysplasiae and is of autosomic dominant transmission; its pathogeny is quite unknown; clinically, it is usually asymptomatic. Rarely arthralgiae of the limbs or concomitant skin anomalies have been described. Usually based on radiological findings, the diagnosis is easy:

- Multiple small bone condensations without changes in the adjacent bone structure
- Electively distributed over the limbs, more seldomly on the shoulder blades and pelvis, very rarely on the spine and the ribs and never on the skull
- Located on the epiphyses and metaphyses of the long bones (metacarpals, phalanges, etc.) or in the central part of the short bones (carpus)
- Most often of rounded configuration, but sometimes forming spots with rather unsharp contours (see the shoulder in case 78)
- Variable number: sometimes a few elements only, sometimes numerous ones
- Time does not alter the appearance. The anomaly, already seen in a child, is still the same in the adult

This 6-year-old child presents with very characteristic morphological changes, permitting a precise diagnosis:

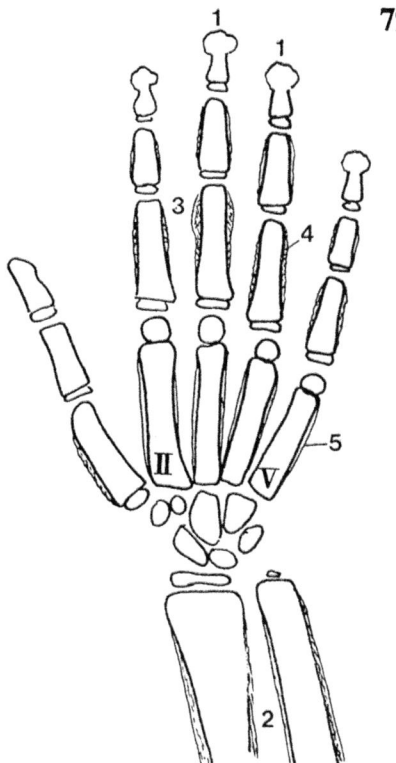

- Hypertrophy of the tuft of the distal phalanges, particularly evident on the third and fourth fingers (*1*) with thickening of the soft parts, especially clear on the thumb. This is a case of digital hippocratism
- Periosteal bone apposition on the diaphyses of the long bones, providing these diaphyses with a fusiform appearance. This is particularly marked on the radius and on the ulna (*2*) and on the proximal phalanges (*3*). The added new cortex can take on an undulating appearance and can thus be clearly distinguished from the ancient cortex (*4*). The neoformed cortex can also be more linear and remain separated for some time from the original cortex by a lucent line (*5*)

The association *digital hippocratism + diaphyseal periosteal appositions* corresponds to *hypertrophic pulmonary osteopathy*. As indicated by its name, these bone changes are secondary to a pneumopathy which can only be chronic. In case 79 the causative agent was mucoviscidosis. As a matter of fact, this is one of the rare causes of chronic respiratory insufficiency in children. Mucoviscidosis usually comprises a polymorphous pulmonary syndrome dominated by a major emphysema.

The evolution of the radiographic changes in hypertrophic pulmonary osteopathy depends on the causative disease. Regression is thus possible. The same anomalies are encountered in the adult, but with predominance of digital hippocratism. The bone anomalies are not proportional to respiratory insufficiency; conversely, they can exist before the pulmonary manifestations and can then be a clue for them.

Hippocratism is still a riddle. There is a long list of diseases in which it can appear: respiratory insufficiency, bronchial cancer, bacterial endocarditis and cyanogenous congenital cardiopathies.

80

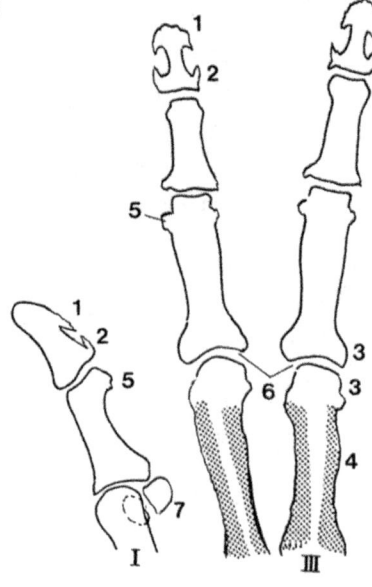

Obviously this adult also exhibits an osteopathy which could be termed "hypertrophic", but this is not of the same type as case 79. Let us first analyse the abnormalities:

- Widening of the tufts of the distal phalanges with bony spurs on the sides (*1*)
- Bony spikes at the base of the distal phalanges, developing in a distal direction (*2*), thus in the opposite direction with regard to the osteophytes
- Widening of the phalangeal and metacarpal heads and bases (*3*)
- Widening of the diaphyses due to periosteal hyperosteogenesis, giving the proximal phalanges and the metacarpals a massive appearance (*4*); cortical thickening without a distinct periosteal lucent line as in hypertrophic pulmonary osteopathy
- Hypertrophy of the crests for ligamentomuscular insertion (*5*)
- Significant widening in the metacarpophalangeal joint spaces (*6*)
- Enlarged sesamoids of the thumb (*7*)

All these changes are consistent with *acromegaly*. The osteoarticular changes in the extremities are among the most typical manifestations of this disease caused by somatotrope pituitary adenoma.

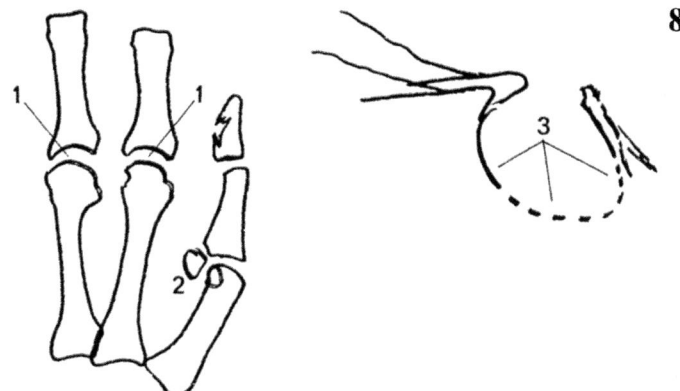

The general configuration of the two hands is also characteristic in this case of *acromegaly*.

Particularly clear here are:
- The enlargement of the metacarpophalangeal joint spaces (*1*) due to hypertrophy of the articular cartilage
- The larger than usual size of the sesamoids on the thumbs (*2*). The sesamoid index (length × width in millimetres) in this disease is 30–60 whereas normally it is below 25.

In more advanced cases, one can see on the hands:
- A paradoxal association of hyperostosis and increased translucency. In fact, periosteal hyperosteogenesis due to proteinic hyperanabolism and a deficient calcic balance called acromegalie osteoporosis coexist
- Non-specific defects in the carpal bones
- Pseudoarthrosic arthropathies due to major osteocartilaginous proliferation.

The roentgen signs on the hands do not occur very early in the history of the disease. The *soft tissue thickening* occurs first and can be measured on the foot sole on a lateral view of the posterior tarsus. Our patient has here a plantar sole thickness of 29 mm while normal values are below 21 mm. A thickness of 23 mm enables the presence of acromegaly to be affirmed.

Since somatotrope adenomas are usually late findings, they are usually macroadenomas measuring over 10 mm. In such cases *destruction of the margins of the sella turcica* and increased size are frequent (*3*). The radiological analysis of the adenoma proper is performed with tomodensitometry.

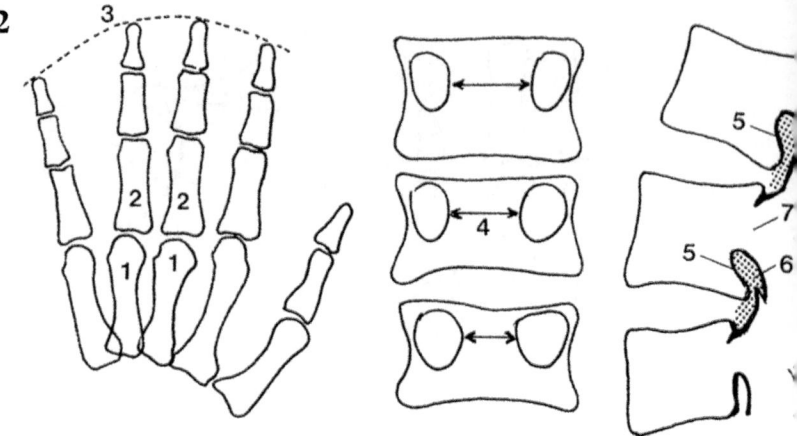

In this patient you will note on the hands:

- Shortening of the second, third and fourth metacarpals, with a somewhat massive appearance of the diaphyses and metacarpal heads (*1*)
- A somewhat short appearance of the phalanges but their general morphology is normal (*2*)
- A globally compact appearance of the hand, the last four fingers having approximately the same length (*3*)
- The right-left symmetry of the above-listed changes

Global shortening of the hands is rarely an isolated finding. Other different structures of the skeleton are usually concerned, in particular the spine. There, the major anomalies are the following:

- Decrease from above downwards in the interpedicular distance (*4*) whereas the contrary is normal
- Anteroposterior shortening in the vertebral bodies due in fact to exaggerated concavity of their posterior aspect (*5*) (scalloping)
- Anteroposterior narrowing of the intervertebral foramina (*6*) due to shortness of the pedicles (*7*)

The diagnosis of *achondroplasia* is made on the association of the following radiological findings: globally shortened fingers + progressive, from above downwards, stenosis of the lumbar canal. Achondroplasia is not the only dysplasia comprising short fingers (acromelia), but all other eventualities are extremely rare and their precise identification is difficult (e.g. pseudo-achondroplasia, spondylo-epiphyso-metaphyseal dysplasia, etc.). There are, besides the skeletal abnormalities, other different malformations that are often associated, which render diagnosis easier, or on the contrary, more complicated.

On the hands of this 9-year-old girl you can see:

- A globally short and compact appearance of the hands
- Irregular contours of most of the carpal bones (*1*) and of the lower radial epiphysis (*2*)
- Irregularities in the metaphyseal limit of the metacarpals (*3*) milder in the phalanges
- Slight irregularity of some metacarpal epiphyses (*4*)
- Cone shape of some of the phalangeal epiphyses (*5*)

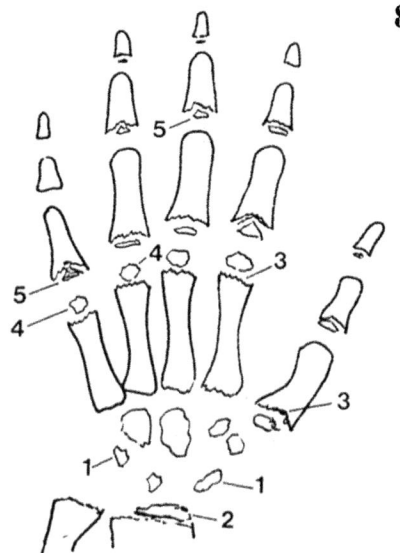

The diagnosis here is relatively difficult. The association acromelia + metaphyseal irregularities leads to the diagnosis of *polyepiphyseal dysplasia*. This condition is recognized at variable ages, most often between 2 and 10 years, sometimes only in the adult. It comprises moderate statural insufficiency, normal skull, often normal spine, shortness of the extremities predominating on hands and feet.

Polyepiphyseal dysplasia belongs to the group of the osteochondrodysplasiae. It is clearly distinct from achondroplasia, which comprises typical craniovertebral changes. It is, however, situated in the larger group of spondyloepiphyso-metaphyseal dysplasiae, in which the classification of the diverse components is still controversial, due to the complexity of the different anomalies.

84

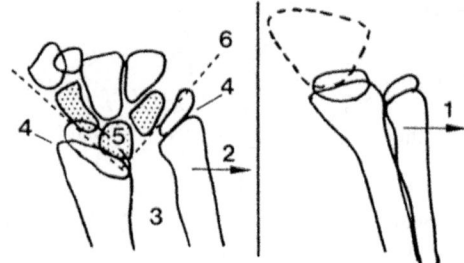

This 10-year-old girl with moderate dwarfism has been X-rayed for bilateral shortening of the forearm with deformity of the wrist. Let us analyse the radiological findings:

- External incurvation of the radius in the frontal plane
- Posterior (*1*) and medial (*2*) luxation of the lower ulnar extremity
- Widening of the interosseous space (*3*)
- Inferior obliquity of the radius and ulna (*4*)
- Ogival carpus (*5*) the tip of which is formed by the lunate wedged into the enlarged radioulnar space. The carpal angle is markedly decreased: 90° (normal, 131° ± 7°) (*6*)

All these changes are characteristic of *Madelung's deformity*. This unaesthetic deformity is usually bilateral, occurs mainly in females, is often familial and is not very disabling.

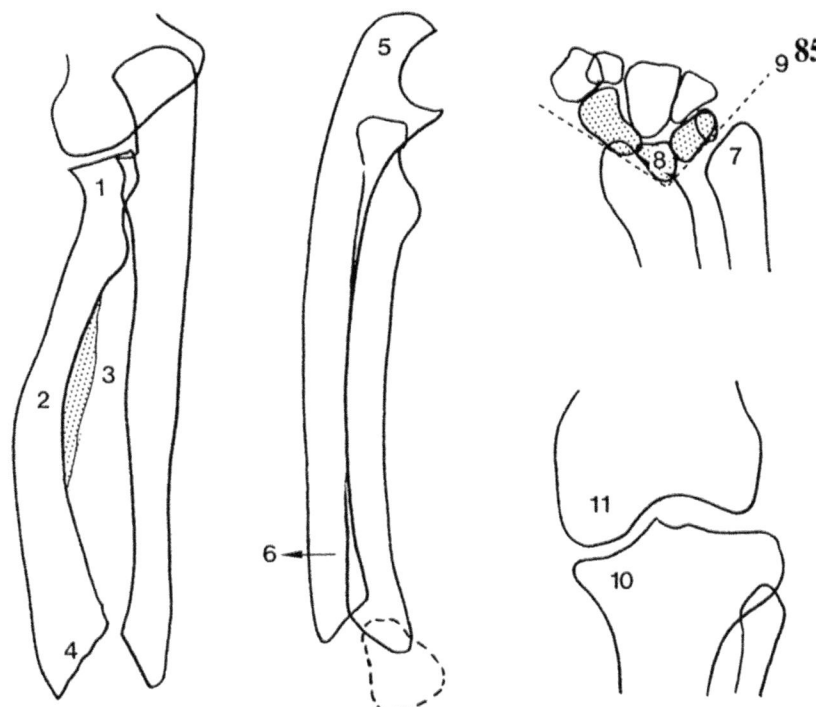

This 16-year-old girl presents the same unaesthetic infirmity of the forearms and wrists. From the radiological point of view, the symptomatology here is much more complete:

– Radial head flattened and slightly hypoplatic (*1*)
– Lateral diaphyseal curvature of the radius (*2*)
– Accentuation of the interosseous crest of the radius (*3*)
– Inferior obliquity of the radius (*4*)
– Bulky appearance of the olecranon (*5*)
– Posteromedial luxation of the lower ulnar extremity (*6*) with lack of modelling (*7*)
– Cup-shaped carpus, with the lunate on the tip (*8*) and a strongly decreased carpal angle measuring 102° (*9*)

The only other skeletal abnormality is a bilateral genu varum by hypoplasia of the medial tibial plate (*10*) compensated by hypertrophy of the medial femoral condyle (*11*).

On the basis of such radiological anomalies, only one diagnosis should be discussed: *dyschondrosteosis or Leri-Weill syndrome.*

According to Maroteaux, dyschondrosteosis and Madelung's deformity represent the same condition. Madelung's deformity, affecting only the forearm and the wrist, is one of the components of dyschondrosteosis. Almost similar radiological changes are found in other malformative variants like Turner's syndrome and multiple exostosis.

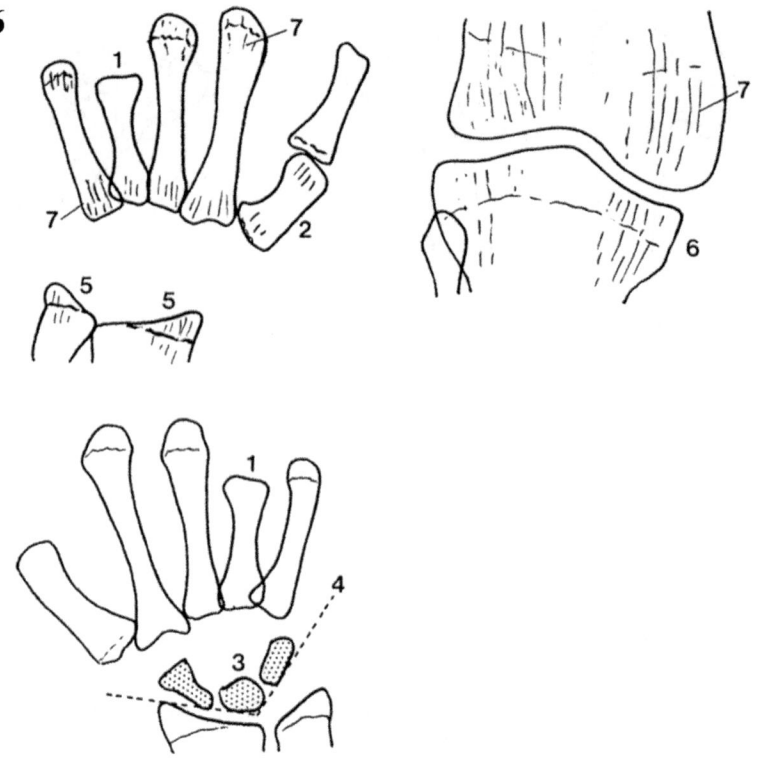

Multiple anomalies can be noted in this 16-year-old girl:

- Brachymetacarpy: fourth digit on both sides (*1*) and first on the left (*2*)
- Ogival wrist, the lunate forming the summit (*3*), the carpal angle being decreased and measuring 115° (*4*)
- Inferior obliquity of the radius and ulna (*5*)
- Brachymetatarsy: third and fourth digits
- Hypoplasia of the medial tibial plate (*6*) compensated for by asymmetrical femoral condyles
- Retardation in the bone age, which was evaluated to be 13 years
- Coarse longitudinal striations in the bone trabeculations of the epiphyses, specially marked on the knee (*7*), less obvious on the hands

The association brachymetacarpy of the fourth finger + hypoplasia of the medial tibial plate is very characteristic for a case of *Turner's syndrome*. It is a chromosomal malformation syndrome with a karyotype comprising 45 chromosomes with only one X: 45 X.

Brachymetacarpy of the first (*1*) and of the fourth (*2*) digit is easy to recognize. Inferior radioulnar obliquity (*3*), a carpal angle reduced to 114° (*4*) and the ogival configuration of the first row of the carpal bones are less evident.

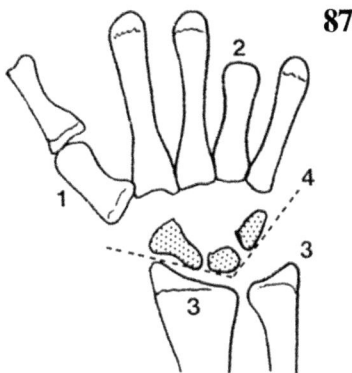

87

This too is a case of *Turner's syndrome*. This chromosomal malformation syndrome comprises ovarian agenesia with subsequent ovarian deficit, causing at puberty an absence of development of the secondary sex characters, short stature, delayed bone maturation, a small sella turcica and different malformations, the most characteristic of which are the association: brachymetacarpy of the fourth finger (Archibald's sign) + hypoplasia of the medial tibial plate (Kosowicz's sign). Turner's syndrome is relatively common. Just as common are incomplete form and other chromosomic variants with partial radiological changes.

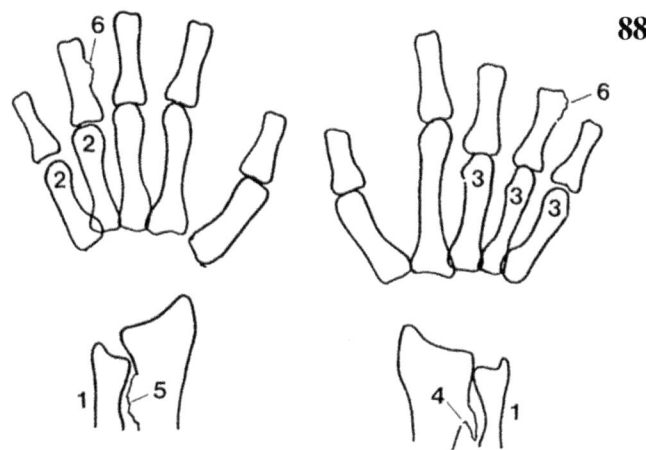

88

Three types of anomalies dominate here:

- Bilateral shortening of the ulna (*1*)
- Shortening of several metacarpals: fourth and fifth on the right hand (*2*) and third, fourth and fifth on the left hand (*3*)
- Multiple exostoses, some pedunculated (*4*), others sessile (*5*), sometimes poorly evident (*6*)

The association exostoses + brachymetacarpy leads to the diagnosis of *multiple exostosis*.

This osteochondrodysplasia, with autosomal dominant inheritance, predominating in males, usually comprises dwarfism, juxta-articular swelling due to metaphyseal exostoses of the long bones and frequent involvements of shoulder blades, pelvis and ribs. Deformity of the wrist is commonly seen. Ulnar shortening is a constant feature with correlative ulnar deviation of the hand. These features are clearly different from those of Madelung's deformity. Exostoses occur and gradually develop in children and young adults. Phalangeal exostoses are frequent but are not always much developed.

89 We shall now see the broad group of the *brachydactylies,* dominated by the *brachymetacarpies.* In case 89 you will have easily recognized the bilateral isolated shortening of the fourth metacarpal.

The term brachydactyly merely designates the shortness of a finger, with no precise indication as to what bone piece is responsible. A more precise denomination permits exact identifications: brachymetacarpy when it is the metacarpal, brachybasophalangy, brachymesophalangy or brachytelephalangy when it is the proximal, middle or distal phalanx, respectively.

Brachydactylies represent numerically the most frequent malformation of the hand and, functionally, are the best tolerated. It is, however, impossible to determine the real frequency since the anomaly is often too subtle to require medical care. From the aetiological point of view, one must distinguish between the acquired and the congenital forms. Usually the acquired forms do not result in any problems, on account of the clinical context and the radiological appearance. This is quite different with the congenital forms.

90 In this next patient you will have also easily identified *congenital brachymetacarpy* of the fifth finger on one side, and of the fourth and fifth fingers on the other side. Among brachydactylies in general, metacarpal involvements are the most frequent.

In practice, one is faced with three types of situation:
- The malformation is isolated or apparently isolated; this is the most frequent case
- It may be evident and associated with differently known and more or less complex malformative syndromes
- It may be initially unrecognized and searched for in the group of diverse malformations known usually to comprise this anomaly; its visualization, especially by X-rays, is a supplementary argument for the diagnosis of its type.

Diverse, more or less complex classifications have been proposed but none makes possible the classification in a simple, rapid and logical way of all the possibilities encountered.

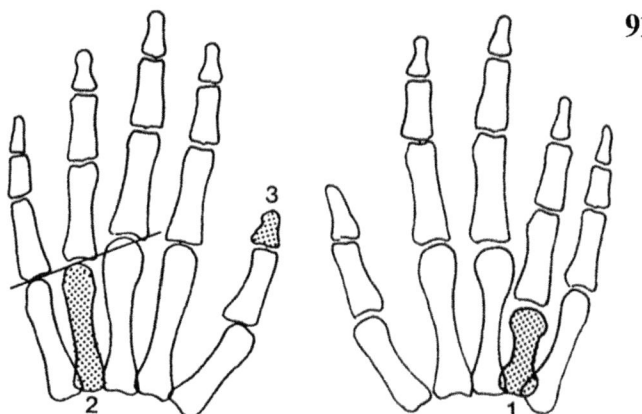

Several abnormalities are obvious in this girl aged 15 years:

– Marked brachymetacarpy of the fourth finger on one side (*1*)
– Much less evident brachymetacarpy of the fourth finger on the other hand (*2*); if we draw the line tangent to the fourth and fifth metacarpal heads, the diagnosis becomes evident
– Brachytelephalangy of the thumb (*3*)

The *fourth metacarpal,* the *distal phalanx of the thumb* and the *middle phalanx of the fifth finger* are elective sites for congenital shortenings. Involvement of the proximal phalanges is exceptional and always associated with other localizations and especially with other malformations. The middle phalanges are more frequently affected, the distal phalanges rarely, except of the thumb. Simultaneous involvement of the feet is rather rare, often not very obvious, being only an aesthetic problem.

Involvement here is really symmetrical:

– Brachymetacarpy of the fifth digit
– Brachytelephalangy of the thumb

The right-left symmetry is indeed very common, but the severity of the involvement often differs.

Brachytelephalangy of the thumb is frequent, often familial, for instance, mother-daughter. Females are moreover more often affected. When the anomaly is unilateral, it always affects the same side in the same family.

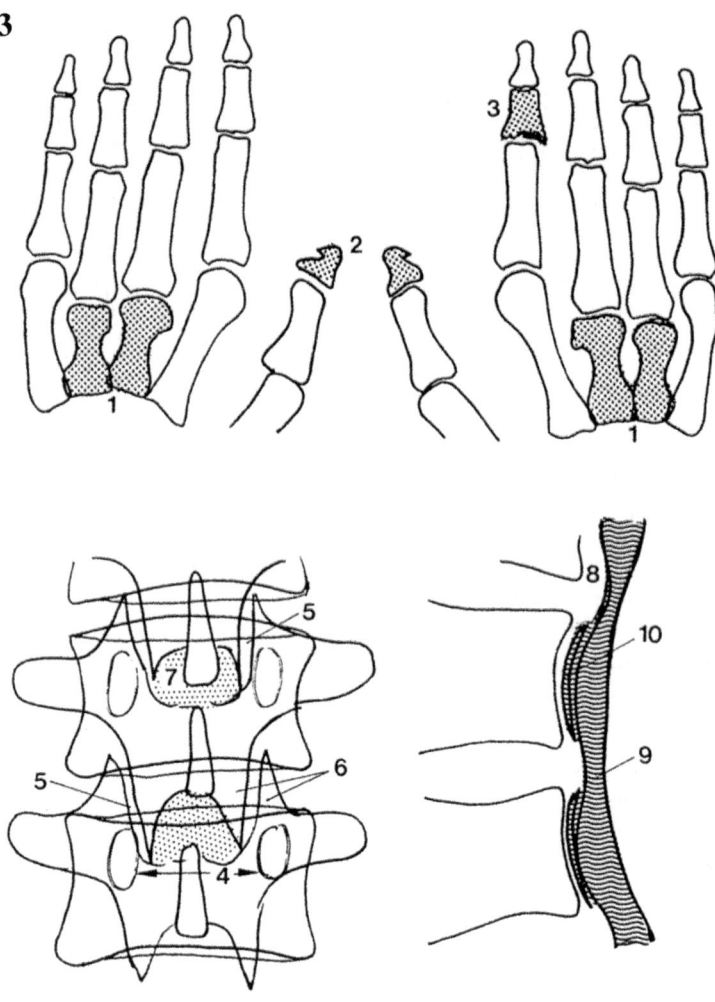

Brachydactylies may be associated with diverse malformative syndromes. In this patient there are numerous and almost symmetrical anomalies of the hands:

– Bilateral brachymetacarpy of the third and fourth metacarpals (*1*). As a result the last four fingers have almost the same length
– Bilateral brachytelephalangy of the thumb (*2*)
– Brachymesophalangy of the second finger on the left. This phalanx is short but also broad, with deformity and irregularity of its proximal extremity, suggesting the pre-existence of a cone-shaped epiphysis (*3*).

This patient moreover has anomalies of the same type on both feet, with multiple brachydactylies. Other characteristic anomalies affect the lumbar spine:

- No increase in the interpediculate distance from above downward (*4*)
- Posterior articular interspaces seen in the sagittal plane (*5*)
- Hypertrophy of the posterior articular processes (*6*)
- Reduction of the interlaminar spaces (*7* – stippled design)
- Narrowing of the intervertebral foramina due to shortening of the pedicles and hypertrophy of the posterior articular processes (*8*)
- Reduced AP diameter of the dural sac (*9*) with retrocorporeal stasis of the contrast medium during radiculosaccography (*10*)

This is thus a case of an association: congenital narrow lumbar canal + multiple brachydactylies, corresponding to *cheirolumbar dysostosis.*

94

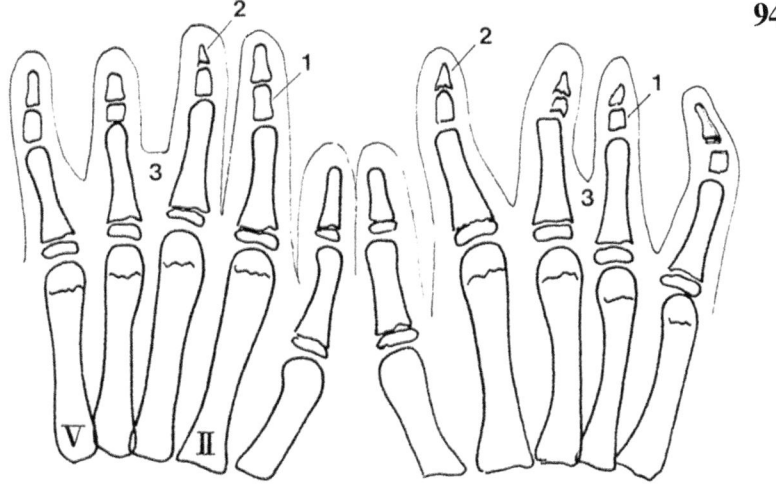

The hands of this 15-year-old boy show:

- Brachymesophalangy of the second and fifth fingers on both hands (*1*)
- Brachytelephalangy of the second, third and fourth fingers on both hands (*2*)
- Different deformities of the hands resulting from the above-listed anomalies
- Syndactyly of the soft parts between several fingers on both sides (*3*)

In this patient, however, the complex malformative appearance of the skull and of the facial skeleton predominates, which enables us to classify this case in the group of the *orodigitofacial syndrome.*

   This is thus an example in which the malformations on the hands, although marked, are only one of the components of a complex dysostosis.

95

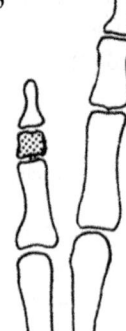

This is a case of bilateral brachymesophalangy on the fifth finger. The anomaly is absolutely identical on both sides. It concerns a 49-year-old man with no other pathological history.

Note, however, that anomalies of the middle phalanx of the fifth finger are frequent:

– Either simple shortening
– Or unequal shortening, more pronounced on the radial than on the ulnar side, causing flexion of the fifth finger towards the fourth; it is a *clinodactyly*. This disorder is often associated with *trisomy 21*.

96

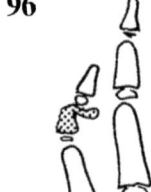

This case represents bilateral *brachyclinodactyly* of the fifth finger of very unusual configuration and real subtotal luxation of the phalangeal head.

97

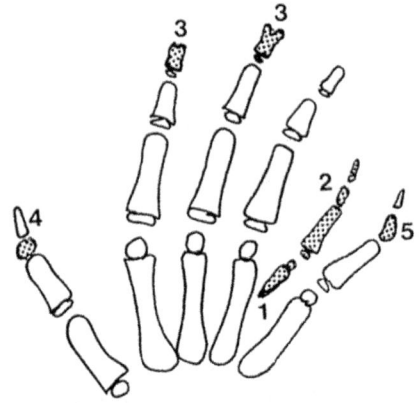

This child with six fingers has *poly-dactyly*. The sixth finger arises between the fourth and fifth; it comprises:

– A rudimentary distal metacarpal (*1*)
– Hypoplastic phalanges (*2*)

Diverse malformative syndromes are seen on the same hand:

– Rudimentary duplication of the distal phalanx of the second and third fingers (*3*)
– On the distal phalanx of the thumb the epiphysis is too voluminous with regard to the rest of the bone piece
– Clinodactyly on the middle phalanx of the fifth finger (*5*)

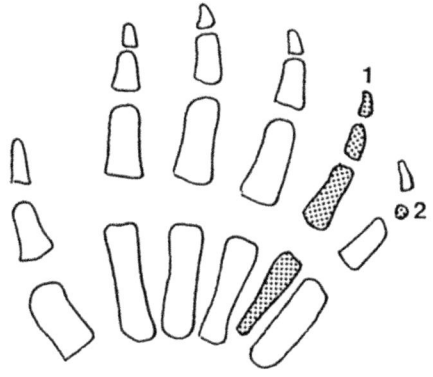

98

This other child also exhibits *polydactyly*. The sixth finger is situated between the fourth and the fifth. It has an almost normal configuration, but all bone elements are somewhat hypoplastic (*1*). Also the middle phalanx of the fifth finger is markedly hypoplastic so that there is brachyclinodactyly (*2*).

In both cases, 97 and 98, polydactyly and the other minor anomalies on the hand are isolated. This is the most frequent case. Polydactyly may, however, be associated with different, more or less complex, malformative syndromes.

Polydactyly comprises usually only one accessory digit, rarely two. Three varieties are to be distinguished:

– Duplication of the thumb, called preaxial polydactyly
– Duplication of the fifth finger, called postaxial polydactyly
– Extra digits at the level of the three median fingers (cases 97 and 98)

Whatever its site, the extra digit is almost always malformed; it may consist of a rudimentary digit without skeleton or of a more or less complete finger. Duplication may occur at the level of the metacarpals, the phalanges, or sometimes only of the distal phalanx. The extra digit can be separated from the others or more or less fused with them, associating polydactyly and syndactyly.

99

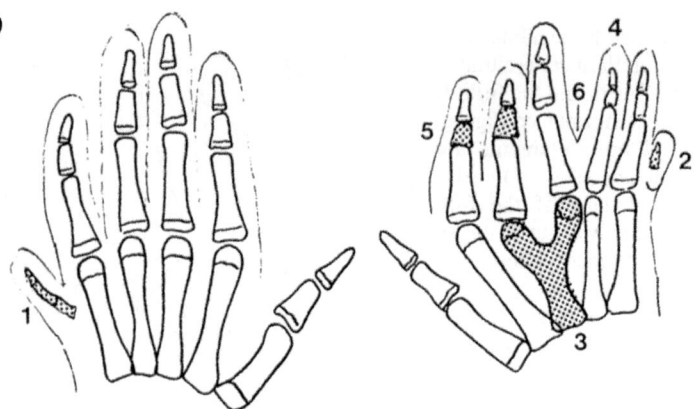

This bizarre polydactyly was seen in a complex malformation syndrome: the *Laurence-Moon-Biedl-Bardet syndrome.*

The radiological findings in the hand are:
- Rudimentary postaxial polydactyly on the fifth metacarpal on the right (*1*)
- Rudimentary postaxial polydactyly on the proximal phalanx of the fifth finger on the left (*2*)
- Duplication of the third left metacarpal (*3*)
- Hypoplasia of all bone elements of the fourth left finger; its total length is the same as the fifth (*4*)
- Apparent shortening of the middle phalanx of the second and third left fingers (*5*) of uncertain pathology, since it could be due to partial flexion of these two digits
- Syndactyly with partial fusion of the soft tissues of almost all fingers of the left hand (*6*)

This child has moreover retinis pigmentosa and psychomotor retardation, so that the diagnosis of Laurence-Moon-Biedl-Bardet syndrome can be considered.

In the presence of polydactyly other different syndromes can also be discussed: the Ulrich-Feichtiger syndrome, acrofacial dysostosis of Weyers, trisomy 13, etc. They have in common that they are rare, very complex and of difficult diagnosis. Polydactyly is only a trivial component of them.

Child's hand with multiple malformations:

- Duplication of the thumb, thus preaxial polydactyly (*1*)
- Triphalangeal thumb with an intermedian piece between the proximal and distal phalanges (*2*)
- Irreducible flexion of the proximal interphalangeal joint of the fifth finger, termed camptodactyly (*3*). Camptodactyly should not be mistaken for clinodactyly of the fifth finger, in which case there is asymmetrically reduced length of the middle phalanx, and thus curvature, and not flexion, of the finger (cases 96 and 97).

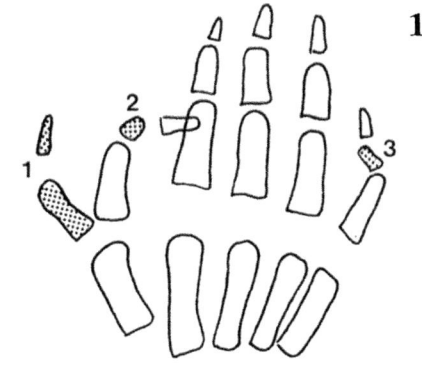

100

Triphalangy of the thumb and *camptodactyly* are seen in diverse malformation syndromes (Holt-Oram syndrome, orodigitofacial syndrome, trisomy 13, etc.). Their diagnosis is always difficult, since the other anomalies can be very complex or, on the contrary, absent or incomplete, depending on diverse combinations.

The malformations here are of two types:

- Postaxial *polydactyly* on the proximal phalanx of the fifth finger (*1*). This extra digit has a rudimentary skeleton
- Syndactyly of the third and fourth fingers (*2*). The digits are more or less fused but the two skeletons remain independent. The syndactyly is more evident since filming was done with the other fingers separate.

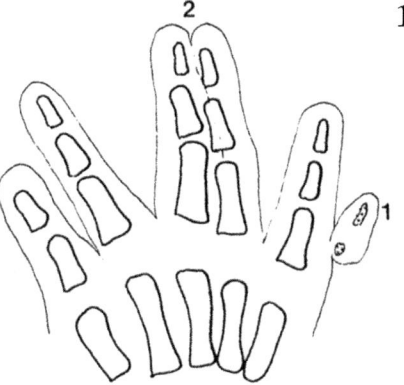

101

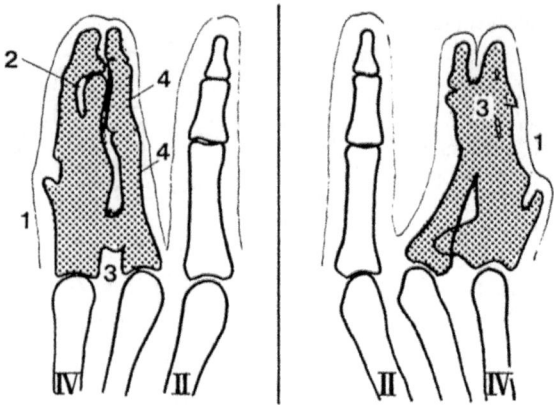

In this case the anomalies are bilateral and affect the third and fourth fingers:

- The phalanges of the fourth finger are hypertrophic, fused, with attempts at articulations (*1*)
- Attempt at duplication of the distal part of the fourth finger (*2*)
- Bony bridges towards the third finger (*3*)
- Thin phalanges on the third finger (*4*)
- Complete coalescence of the soft tissues of the two fingers

This is thus an example of major *syndactyly*. Syndactyly, i.e. fusion of two or several digits, usually concerns the median fingers (second, third, fourth). The malformation can be uni- or bilateral, isolated or associated with other malformations. Simultaneous involvement of the toes is rare. Three degrees of severity can be distinguished:

- Simple cutaneous webbing or synechia
- Fusion of the fingers, with independent skeletons and intact articulations
- More or less complex bone fusion, usually accompanied by tendinous and vasculonervous anomalies, which render surgery difficult

Whatever the type of the malformation, this can be rather proximal to the interdigital commissure, or rather distal with an above-lying commissure, or also, as in case 102, complex and involving the entire digital axis.

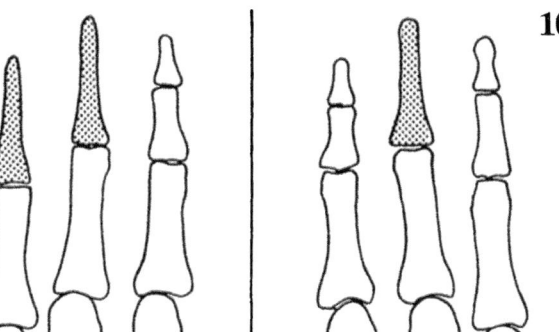

In this patient you will note three distal localizations of *symphalangism*. Fusion of one phalanx to another within the same digit, symphalangism is thus distinct from syndactyly. It is usually inherited as a dominant trait and often unrecognized since it is functionally well tolerated. Depending on the degree of fusion, two varieties are distinguished:

- Complete, with no attempt at articular interspace and with a unique common medullar canal (case 103)
- Incomplete, with all possible intermediate forms, from the vestigial interspace mimicking joint narrowing, to fusion limited to the epiphyses, with independent medullar canals. The diagnosis is easy: there is no cutaneous flexion fold, and the articulation is clinically stiff.

According to the site, symphalangy is said to be:
- Distal, usually isolated (case 103)
- Proximal, often associated either with other malformations on the hand (brachydactyly, etc.) or other synostoses (carpus, tarsus, stapes with oval window), or with complex malformation syndromes (diastrophic dwarfism, Apert's syndrome, etc.).

Note also that the thumb is never affected.

The anomaly you should have identified here is strictly identical on both sides. It is a *synostosis between the trapezoid and the capitate.*

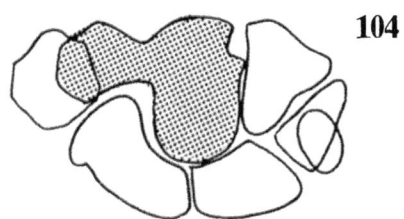

104

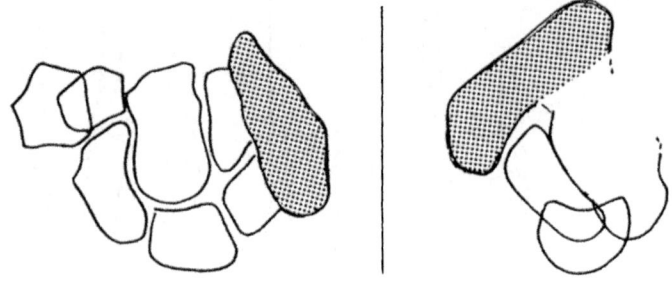

Here two carpal views have facilitated the diagnosis: it is a *pisiform-hamate fusion.*

Carpal fusions are not very common, but their real frequency is certainly underrated since they are usually not symptomatic. The term carpal fusion is probably inadequate, since from the physiopathological point of view the anomaly represents a failure of segmentation of the primitive cartilaginous carpals.

Two variants are distinguished:
- Transverse fusions, involving two bones of the same row (case 104). These localizations are usually isolated, sometimes bilateral. The most frequent is the triquetrum-lunate fusion. Rarer are the capitate-hamate and the trapezium-trapezoid fusions (difficult to affirm because of partial overlap of these bones)
- Longitudinal fusions, i.e. fusion of a bone of the proximal row with a bone of the distal row (case No. 105). The most frequent variety here is the scaphoid-trapezium fusion. Longitudinal fusions are much uncommoner than transverse fusions and are frequently associated with malformation syndromes (Ellis-van Creveld syndrome, arthrogryposis, tarsal fusions, etc.)

Carpal fusions involving more than two bones are extremely rare and always symptomatic of multiple malformations.

The *complexity of the malformations* on the hand has no limits. Note in this child:

– Syndactyly of the second and third fingers (*1*)
– Aplasia of the distal phalanx of the second, third and fourth fingers
– Symphalangism of the third finger (*2*)
– On the second finger, an epiphyseal nucleus in the distal phalanx very close to the proximal phalanx developing subsequent partial symphalangism (*3*). This joint is not functional because of the syndactyly and the adjacent symphalangism
– Brachyclinodactyly of the fifth finger (*4*)

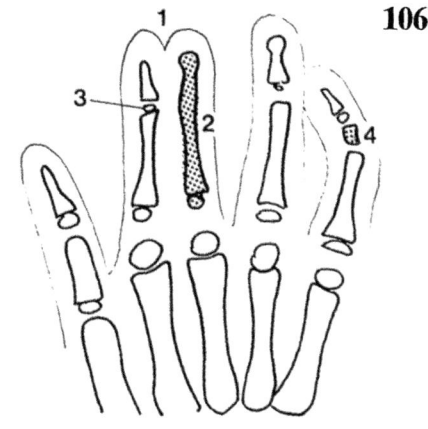

106

In this other child, agenesia is transverse and distal:

– Agenesis of the distal phalanx of the thumb
– Agenesis or very severe hypoplasia of the middle and distal phalanges of the other fingers (*1*)
– Abnormal broadening of the proximal phalanx of the thumb and of the index (*2*)

Cases 106 and 107 represent distal variants of *terminal aplasiae*. Here they are *aphalangies*. Absence of digits, or adactyly, and absence of hand, or acheiria, are severe forms of terminal aplasiae.

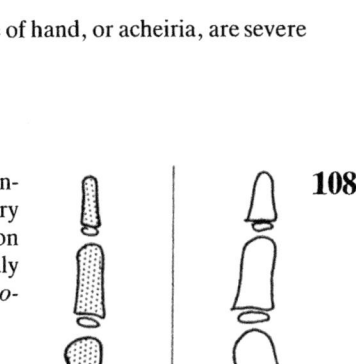

107

All phalangeal or digital *hypoplasiae* are not congenital. In this 5-year-old child, there is very clearly hypotrophy of the thumb, by comparison with the unaffected side. In this case the anomaly results from and is a sequel of *infantile encephalopathy*.

108

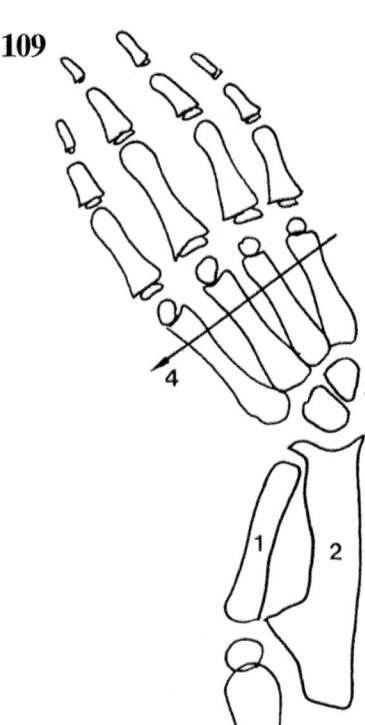

109

This 8-year-old child has a complex malformation of the upper limb:

- Hypoplasia of the radius (*1*) and ulna (*2*) with luxation of the elbow
- Only two carpal bones, probably the capitate and the hamate (*3*)
- Absence of the thumb
- Deviation of the hand towards the radius, called radial club hand (*4*)

This child has also been operated on at birth for oesophageal atresia and has other, extra-skeletal, malformations.

Absence of the thumb, absence of the radial aspect of the carpus and hypoplasia predominant on the radius lead to classification of this malformation in the group of the *radial ray aplasiae*. There are also aplasiae of the ulnar ray and of the median rays: they all belong to the general group of *longitudinal aplasiae*.

Absence of the thumb can be seen in some syndromes, such as Werner's syndrome and occasionally the Holt-Oram syndrome. ¯

Child, aged 3 years, with a voluminous middle finger:

– Moderately hypertrophic metacarpal (*1*)
– Enlargement of the phalanges in all their dimensions, but more in the width than in the length (*2*)
– Particularly enlarged tuft of the distal phalanx (*3*)
– Advanced bone age with regard to the other fingers, i.e. the epiphyseal centres are not only more developed, but this of the distal phalanx is present and large, whereas it is lacking on the adjacent fingers (*4*)
– Marked hypertrophy of the soft tissues over the affected finger (*5*)

It is thus a case of *macrodactyly,* i.e. hypertrophy of the skeleton and of the soft tissues on one or several digits.

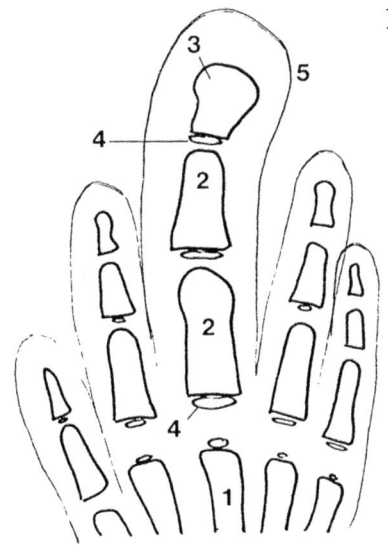

This next child, aged 3 months, also has macrodactyly of the third finger. The radiological findings are the same as in the previous case.

Macrodactyly is a congenital, non-hereditary malformation. It is one of the rarest malformations on the hand, and is almost always isolated. It is even rarer on the toes. There are two varieties of macrodactyly:

– Static: the enlargement of the finger is present at birth, but its development occurs proportionally with the other fingers
– Progressive: development occurs at a faster rate, and the finger increases more and more in size with regard to the other fingers. In case 110, the bone age is advanced with regard to the other fingers, so that one can foresee a progressively faster growth with regard to the unaffected fingers

In any case, growth of the affected finger stops together with the global growth arrest of the skeleton. The sites described in the literature are almost always the second and the third fingers, never the thumb. Simultaneous involvement of two fingers is more frequent (50%) than of one (35%). Different pathogenic hypotheses have been considered. In any case it is a congenital neuroectodermic dysplasia, so that macrodactyly is thus related to phacomatoses. The preferential involvement of the second and third fingers suggests a process concerning the median nerve. *Neurofibromatosis of Recklinghausen* seems the best aetiological hypothesis.

112

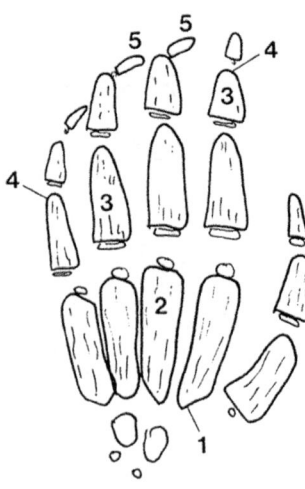

Different anomalies must have been recognized on the hands of this 6-year-old child:

- The proximal ends of the metacarpals have a pointed appearance, particularly evident on the second and third fingers (*1*)
- Enlargement of the medulla and thinning of the cortex of the metacarpals (*2*) and of the phalanges, which have a short and trapezoidal appearance (*3*)
- The distal ends of the proximal and middle phalanges are rounded (*4*)
- The distal phalanges are hypoplastic and have a clawlike configuration
- Delayed bone maturation

Further skeletal anomalies (enlargement of the ribs, scaphocephaly due to premature closure of the sagittal suture, anterosuperior aplasia of a vertebral body in the thoracolumbar joint) and extraskeletal changes (facial dysmorphy, macroglossy, psychomotor retardation) associated with the very characteristic changes on the hands lead to the diagnosis of *Hurler's syndrome* or *mucopolysaccharidosis I.*

113

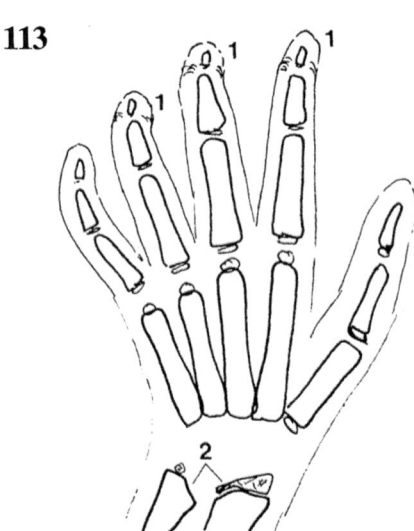

Two anomalies, identical on both sides, are the only skeletal changes in this 8-year-old child:

- Claw-like deformity of the distal phalanges (*1*)
- Inferior radioulnar obliquity (*2*)

Associated with moderate dwarfism and clouding of the cornea, these very characteristic anomalies on the hands lead to the diagnosis of *Ullrich-Scheie's disease* or *mucopolysaccharidosis V.*

Mucopolysaccharidoses, of which there are at present about ten different types, are hereditary disturbances in the metabolism of the mucopolysaccharides. This enzymatic insufficiency is responsible for enchondral growth disturbances.

In this man aged 32 years, the radiography of the hand was performed to determine bone age, because of pituitary disturbances. You will have certainly noticed the persistent growth cartilage. The radiograph shows moreover:

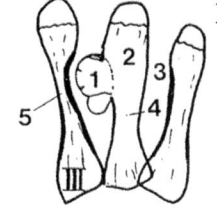

114

- A bilobated expansion on the radial aspect of the diaphysis of the fourth metacarpal, with onset of septations within the expansion (*1*)
- The diaphysis of this metacarpal is poorly modelled, with a club-shaped deformity of its distal end (*2*)
- Marked thinning of the cortex (*3*)
- Very poor bone structure in the medulla (*4*)
- Thinning of the adjacent third metacarpal, with reactional thickening of the cortical bone (*5*)

This is obviously a *benign tumour,* already long-standing as is proved by the imprint and the cortical reaction on the adjacent metacarpal. The radiological findings lead us to discuss two diagnoses:

- Chondroma
- Osteochondroma or osteocartilaginous exostosis

The first diagnosis is chosen, since osteochondroma is rarely located on the hands (rather on the humerus or on the femur) and also because its contour is more irregular and the centre more dense and heterogeneous.

This is obviously a lesion similar to the previous one, although less advanced, arising from the cortical and subcortical region on the fourth metacarpal. Note also:

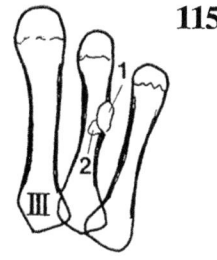

115

- Slight bulging of the cortex (*1*)
- Centromedullary expansion (*2*)

The *chondroma is the commomest tumour of the hand.* It is encountered equally in males and females, at any age, but with a clear predominance in the young adult. Two main circumstances lead to its radiological diagnosis: slowly progressive and painless swelling, or a chance finding when the patient is X-rayed after a trauma.

The sites usually affected are the metacarpals and proximal and middle phalanges; more rarely involved is the thumb, exceptionally the distal phalanges and almost never the carpus. The chondroma is usually located on the diaphysis, either in the middle part or adjacent to the metaphysis.

116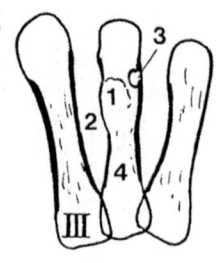

Note on this fourth metacarpal:

- A defect situated somewhat eccentrically towards the lateral margin of the diaphysis (*1*); its medial limits are unsharp, but somewhat better defined on a tomogram
- Thinning and mild fusiform bulging of the cortex (*2*)
- Microdefect under the ulnar aspect of the metaphyseal region (*3*) with a mild medial alteration of the cortex. This second defect seems totally independent of the main localization
- A somewhat trabeculated appearance of the diaphyseal medulla (*4*)

The diagnosis is *chondroma*. From the radiological point of view two varieties of chondroma of the skeleton of the hand can be distinguished:

- *Enchondroma* (case 116). The lucent defect is intraosseous, rounded or polycyclic with more or less well-defined margins. Septations are uncommon. Intratumoral calcifications are exceptional. The cortex may be thinned on its medial aspect and expanded
- *Juxtacortical chondroma* (cases 114 and 115). This develops within or beneath the periosteum. The cortex may be:
  - Expanded from inside outwards when the lesion develops within or directly beneath the cortex.
  - Eroded from outside inwardly, with an osteosclerotic margin on the side of the medullar cavity, when the lesion develops at the level of the periosteum.

117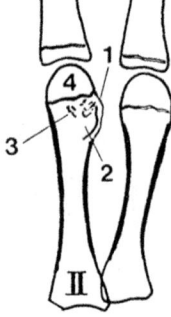

The diagnosis of *chondroma* on the hand varies in difficulty: it is most often easy; occasionally, however, it is much less evident. In this girl, aged 16 years, without local symptomatology, the changes on the second metacarpal are still very discreet:

- Slight expansion of the juxtametaphyseal cortex (*1*)
- Juxtametaphyseal defect with unsharp limits (*2*)
- Small calcifications within and in the neighbourhood of the defect (*3*)
- Unremarkable epiphyses and growth cartilage (*4*). As long as the growth cartilage is present, the epiphysis is unaffected.

Unlike in the previous case, the diagnosis of *enchondroma* is much more evident here:

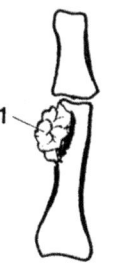

118

- Diaphyseal defect with sometimes regular, sometimes unsharp contours, in the middle part of the phalanx with expansion towards the distal part (*1*)
- Trabeculated appearance of the defect, due to partial septationing
- Circular expansion of the cortex and erosion of its medial aspect (*2*)

Development of chondromas is certainly *very slow*, and very likely some of them remain stationary from a certain time of their evolution on. Often radiographs taken at 2 or 3 years interval show no modifications.

Developmental arrest is also responsible for the fact that the size of the chondromas is usually quite moderate. Juxtacortical chondromas are diagnosed earlier, since they cause dysfunction. The only complication which may occur is the fracture; this is rare, however, even in some strongly exuberant formations.

This *juxtacortical chondroma* on the proximal phalanx of the fourth finger comprises:

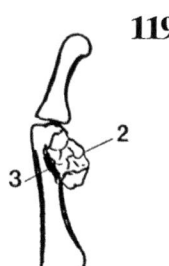

119

- Multiseptate bone mass on the palmar and lateral aspect of the distal part of the diaphysis (*1*)
- Sharp superficial contour (*2*). Note that the soft tissues are still normal
- Slightly densified deep contour (*3*)

This *enchondroma* of the middle phalanx of the second finger is also characteristic (compare with case 118)

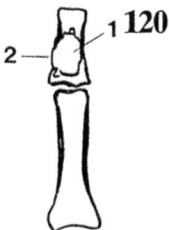

120

- Diaphyseal and basal defect, with regular margin and the beginning of septation (*1*)
- Small localized expansion of the cortex and medial subcortical erosions (*2*)

121

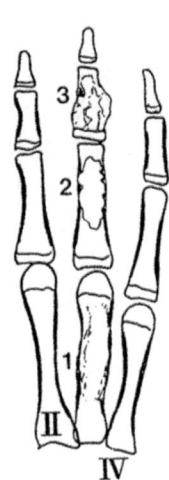

All involvements are situated on the third finger:

– Centrodiaphyseal enchondroma on the metacarpal, with modelling failures in the diaphysis, subcortical erosion and slightly unsharp margins on the ends (*1*)
– Centrodiaphyseal enchondroma of the proximal phalanx, with multiple partial septations, moderate thickening of the diaphysis and subcortical erosions (*2*)
– Enchondroma occupying a major part of the middle phalanx, apart from the ends. Unsharp limits and expansion of the cortex (*3*)

Usually the chondroma is isolated. As soon as there are multiple locations, a fortiori when they are unilateral, the diagnosis of *enchondromatosis or Ollier's disease* must be considered.

Ollier's disease, formerly called dyschondroplasia of Ollier, classically has a mainly unilateral distribution. This is a syndrome of multiple enchondromas, equally frequently located on the pelvis, the shoulder blades and the long bones of the limbs. The severity of the disease is very variable. Some patients have only rare, well-tolerated involvements. The severe forms are associated with shortening of the affected limbs. The risk of sarcomatous degeneration is rather high: about 30%, but concerns mainly the proximal and axial sites (scapula, vertebra, etc.). There are various opinions concerning the pathogeny: embryopathy, recessive hereditary disorder, not transmissible genetic mutation.

122

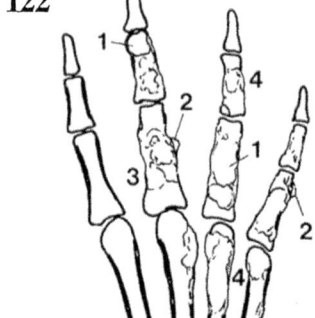

This manual worker, aged 44 years, X-rayed because of a trivial trauma to the hand, shows multiple localizations of chondromatous appearance; the first two fingers and the distal phalanges are uninvolved. There are four types of anomalies:

– Intraosseous defects (*1*)
– Juxta- and intracortical defects (*2*)
– Condensing and microlacunar mixed dystrophy, predominantly on the proximal phalanges (*3*)
– Slightly irregular deformity of the cortices, mainly producing a failure in the modelling of the diaphyses (*4*)

Three diagnoses must be discussed:

- *Fibrous dysplasia:* localization on several bones, disorders in the modelling of the diaphyses, and the mixed, lacunar and condensing, changes on almost all affected bones are clues in favour of this first diagnosis
- *Maffucci's syndrome:* it is a congenital mesodermic anomaly which associates intra- and extra-osseous chondromatous processes, predominating on the phalanges, with angiomatous tumours with phleboliths. The risk of degeneration of the chondromas here is 20%. The occurrence and rapid multiplication of the involvements during the growth period usually enable an early diagnosis to be made
- *Ollier's disease:* this is the diagnosis which was made. The remaining skeleton in this patient was normal.

This 42-year-old man has a swelling at the base of the index, which had grown rapidly in a few weeks.

123

The radiological findings are alarming:
- Large expansive mass, multilacunar, partially septated, expanding and occupying the phalanx almost totally (*1*)
- Extensively broken cortex (*2*)
- Typically malignant invasion of the soft tissues (*3*) by thin trabeculations of newly formed bone
- Considerable swelling of the soft parts (*4*)
- The metacarpophalangeal joint is spared
- Demineralization of the entire digital axis (*5*)

Since this is obviously a malignant process, we must consider the malignant variety that most commonly involves the hand, i.e. the *chondrosarcoma*. In case 123, it is degeneration of an isolated chondroma, which is an uncommon event. In fact chondrosarcoma is much more often subsequent to known Ollier's disease and, there, it is much more the proximal involvements which have a tendency to degenerate.

124

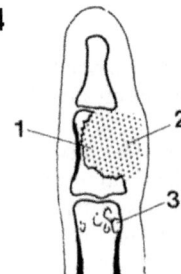

This tumour on the middle phalanx of the second finger also has a frankly malignant character:

- Loss of bone substance affecting a great part of the phalanx, with irregular and unsharp contour (*1*)
- Swelling of the adjacent soft tissues (*2*)
- Small osteolytic lesions in the head of the proximal phalanx (*3*)

This 48-year-old man has a history of bronchial cancer with several secondary osteolytic lesions about the skeleton. There is no doubt as to the diagnosis: *metastasis*.

Metastatic lesions on the hand bones are astonishingly rare, even in particularly polyosseous forms such as epithelioma of the breast. It is almost exclusively bronchial cancer which is responsible for metastases to the hands.

125

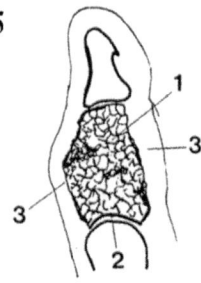

The swelling of the thumb in this 45-year-old man had been recognized for about 5 years. From the only radiological findings, benignity is likely but not certain:

- Lucent defect with multiple septations, entirely occupying the proximal phalanx of the thumb (*1*)
- Only the basal subchondral bone is unaffected (*2*)
- Deformity and expansion, sometimes slightly irregular, of the cortices (*3*) but without rupture and without invasion of the soft tissues. There is a general deformity of the bone piece.

We know that chondromas do not usually involve the thumb, that they leave the epiphysis unaffected and that intratumoral septations are rather uncommon. Since the radiological diagnosis is not categorical, pathological control is necessary. The biopsy diagnosis was *enchondroma*.

126

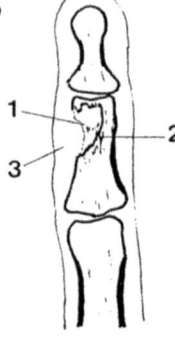

This 31-year-old man had been operated on 5 years previously for a small tumour of the soft tissues, without bone reaction. This local recurrence now comprises bone involvement:

- Slightly irregular lucent defect on the ulnar palmar aspect of the distal part of the middle phalanx (second finger) (*1*)
- Minor sclerotic reaction surrounding the defect (*2*)
- Swelling of the adjacent soft parts (*3*)

It was definitely diagnosed as: *giant cell tumour of the tendon sheath* (flexor sheath).

For 6 months this 29-year-old man had had a swelling on the middle portion of the fourth finger. We note the following changes:

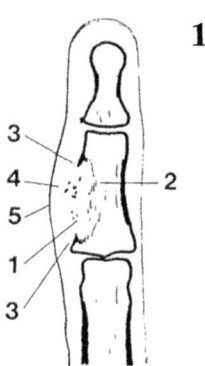

127

- Extended loss of substance on the entire ulnar and palmar aspect of the diaphysis (*1*)
- Fairly irregular limits between the lesion and the normal bone (*2*)
- Spikes on the ends of the substance loss (*3*)
- Microcalcifications within the defect and in the soft tissues (*4*)
- Thickening of the adjacent soft parts (*5*)

It was definitely diagnosed as *giant cell tumour of the tendon sheath* (flexor sheath).

Again this is a proximal phalanx of the fourth finger with an alarming, fairly extended defect (*1*). The limits of the osteolyses are, however, rather well defined (*3*). It also extends towards the base and comes into contact with the joint (*3*).

The diagnosis was: *fibrohistiocytoma of the tendon sheats*.

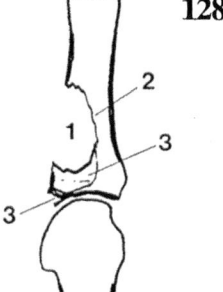

128

This 26-year-old woman has had a painless swelling around the palmar aspect of the third finger, at the level of the first phalanx. A first radiograph had been taken 6 years earlier for the same symptomatology. It had been negative: there had been neither diagnosis nor treatment. Now, 6 years later, the tumefaction is slightly larger but still painless.

The periphery of the tumour is calcified in a smooth way (*1*). There is no bone reaction, but there is a slight deformity of the phalanx over the calcification (*2*). The pathological diagnosis was benign *tumour of the tendon* with cartilaginous metaplasia. On account of its location, it involves the flexor tendon sheath.

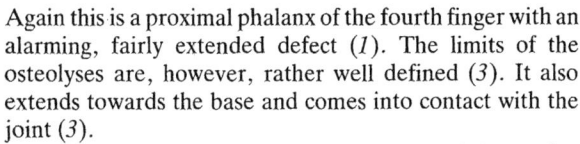

129

Tumours of the tendon sheaths, in particular *giant cell tumour of flexor tendon sheaths,* are relatively common. Bone involvement is always secondary and delayed; it is due to contiguity. The bone reaction is lytic and can have a benign (case 126) or malignant appearance (cases 127 and 128). Bone involvement is not the rule (case 129). The lesion may or may not calcify. Evolution is always fairly long. This type of tumour is benign but often recurrent.

130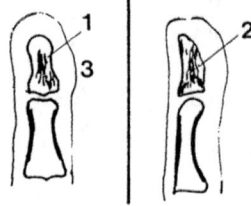

This 16-year-old girl has pain and moderate swelling about the extremity of the third finger. The lesions of this distal phalanx are difficult to analyse:

- Remodelling of the bone structure with alternating condensed areas and ill-delineated microdefects (*1*)
- Slight expansion on the palmar aspect of the bone (*2*)
- No periosteal reaction
- Slight thickening of the soft parts (*3*)

The presence of pain leads us to consider a glomic tumour or osteoid osteoma. The radiological findings do not allow us to conclude, but only to affirm, the benign character of the lesion. It was definitely diagnosed as *osteoid osteoma*.

Apart from chondromas, true primary bone tumours are exceedingly rare on the hands and particularly on the carpus.

131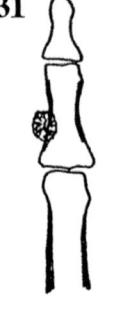

Slight swelling around the medial aspect of the middle of the third finger was present for 1 year in this 55-year-old woman. We note:

- A rounded calcification, measuring 6 mm, slightly heterogeneous, with somewhat irregular contours, in the anteromedial soft tissues of the finger
- Absence of reaction in the adjacent bone; the adjacent phalanx has a normal configuration

Only exeresis could provide the diagnosis: *calcified epidermoid cyst.*

"Calcified tumours" in the soft parts of the fingers are unique, unlike the calcium deposits (Thibierge-Weissenbach syndrome, etc.) and the phleboliths (haemangioma). Tumours only calcify after several years and then remain stationary. They correspond to a limited number of aetiologic varieties: epidermoid cyst (case 131), tumour of the tendon and aponeuroses (case 129), xanthoma and para-articular chondroma.

Referred for rheumatoid arthritis, without hand involvement, this 67-year-old woman has an abnormal but painless distal phalanx of the third finger:

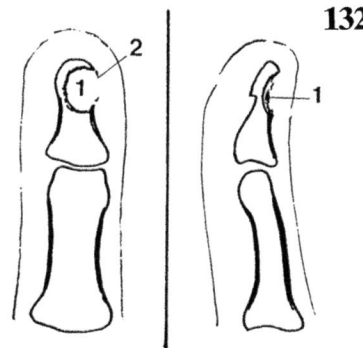

132

- Rounded, homogeneous defect, with sharp and slightly sclerotic contours, on the medial dorsal aspect of the phalangeal extremity (*1*)
- Slight erosion on the lateral aspect of the tuft (*2*)

This is an *epidermoid cyst*. It is a lesion caused by traumatic inclusions of epidermal tissue (needle prick). Its formation takes several years and it may calcify. It is thus not a real "tumour".

This 58-year-old woman had pain around the extremity of her third finger for 15 years which was triggered and exacerbated by touch and cold.

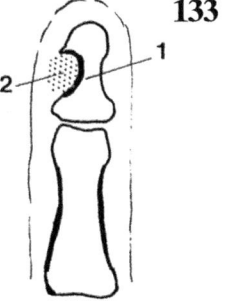

133

The radiological changes are discreet but characteristic:
- Lateral defect on the radial aspect of the distal phalanx; the contours are regular and there is a sclerotic reaction of the cortex (*1*)
- Small rounded mass, faintly visible in the soft parts over the bone defect (*2*)

The association: pain resulting from thermic changes + central or marginal bone erosion compels us to make the diagnosis of *periungual glomus tumour*.

134

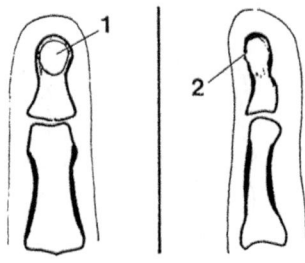

The extremity of the index of this young adult is painful to cold and compression.

The defect developed in the centre of the tuft (*1*) of the distal phalanx is quite characteristic of *glomus tumours*. The slight rupture in the cortex of the dorsal margin (*2*) has no particular significance. The soft parts are unremarkable.

Epidermoid cyst and *glomus tumour or haemangiopericytoma* are the two lesions which electively involve the distal phalanx. The epidermoid cyst is caused by implantation of epidermal tissue in the bone. The lesions being initially intraosseous, the radiograph will show a rounded defect with well-defined and slightly dense contours. The cortex is first intact, but it will be expanded and then rapidly ruptured, depending on the initial site. Later the lesion develops in the soft parts. Being *painless,* it will only be diagnosed at that time.

The glomus tumour or haemangiopericytoma results from the hyperplastic development and the multiplication of the different elements which constitute a normal glomus. The normal glomus is a dermiepidermal arteriovenous anastomosis which plays the role of direct shunt, making temperature control possible. There are numerous glomi in the nailbed and in the fingertips. *Pain* is a constant symptom in glomus tumours. The radiological appearance depends on the site: intraosseous defect at the level of the tuft (case 134), asymmetry of the tuft, which is partly amputated, and notch on the lateral aspect of the phalanx, with a regular and dense contour (case 133).

The radiological appearance of both types of lesions, epidermoid cyst and glomus tumour, can thus be perfectly identical. It is the absence or the presence of pain which helps to differentiate them. Of course, when an arteriography has been performed, the glomus tumour will be characterized by the increased calibre of the collateral artery and by localized hypervascularization with early venous back flow.

This 55-year-old woman has consulted for diffuse pain in the hand of the arthrosic type. The swelling about the middle phalanx of the second finger has existed since her childhood and was considered a sequel of trauma.

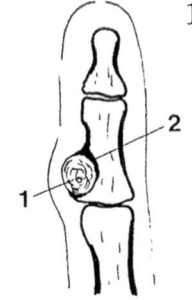

135

The radiograph shows a rounded, stratified calcification, developed in the cortex near the phalangeal base (*1*). A sclerotic margin has formed on a part of its boundary with the medulla (*2*).

Two diagnoses must be discussed:

- *Epidermoid cyst:* all intermediate configurations are possible from the epidermal inclusion only in the soft part with delayed calcification (case 131) or in the bone proper, with constitution of an intraosseous lacuna (case 132)
- *Juxtacortical chondroma,* with intraperiosteal development. This is the most probable diagnosis.

This 23-year-old woman has a hard tumefaction on the cubital aspect of the hand. It has existed for several years without changing.

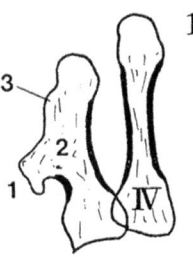

136

Note:

- A bone outgrowth with regular margins, with a large base arising on the middle portion of the ulnar aspect of the fifth metacarpal (*1*)
- Within the outgrowth, a structure identical to the medullar bone of the adjacent diaphysis (*2*)
- Enlargement of the distal end of the diaphysis with a thinned cortex (*3*)

The diagnosis is *osteocartilaginous exostosis* or solitary osteochondroma.

A peculiar form is subungual exostosis; it arises from the tuft of the distal phalanx. Its size usually remains small and does not change. This variety can be considered a mere normal variant.

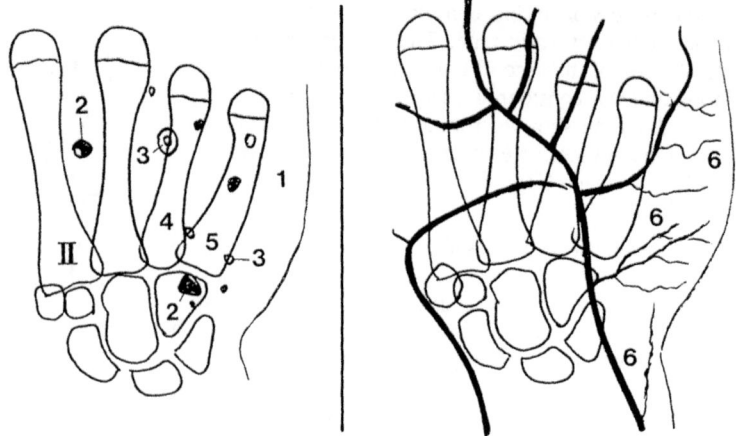

This 10-year-old boy has a non-evolutive, soft swelling on the hand.

The initial radiograph shows:
– Thickening of the soft parts mainly over the ulnar aspect of the hand (*1*)
– Multiple calcifications in the soft tissues: they are of unequal size, some of them highly dense (*2*), others with a centre that is less dense than the periphery (*3*). They are obviously *phleboliths*
– Brachymetacarpy of the fourth finger (*4*)
– Curvature of the fifth metacarpal with abnormal enlargement of the proximal half of its diaphysis (*5*). These bony changes must be considered as trophic disturbances.

Arteriography confirms the diagnosis of *haemangioma:*
– Benign neovascularization, especially in the soft parts of the hypothenar eminence, from the ulnar artery (*6*)

The most characteristic feature is the presence of phleboliths. They permit positive diagnosis, even before angiography.

These are several cases, all of them comprising *juxta-articular ossification or calcification*. This is rather a common eventuality, and several aetiologies must be considered. There are no accessory bones on the fingers, besides the sesamoids. Diagnostic discussion thus concerns:

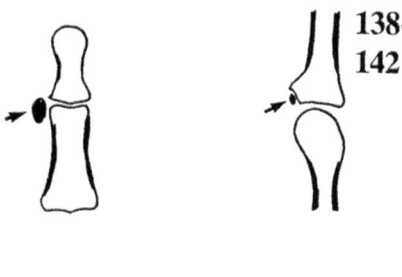

1. *Sequel of Thiemann's disease* (cases 139, 140, 141), i.e. sequel of growth osteochondrosis. The ossicle can be situated in a notch on the base of the phalanx (cases 139 and 141) or freely adjacent to the joint
2. *Traumatic avulsion* (case 142). When the trauma is recent, the fracture line is usually easily recognized (see case 28). Long-standing avulsion is, however, difficult to affirm. Case 142 is interesting insofar as the radiograph has

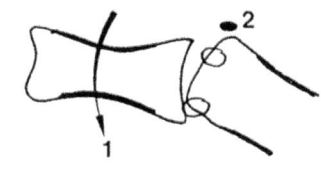

been taken in a stress position, i.e. forced abduction, which produces subluxation (by ligamentous laxity or rupture) of the proximal phalanx of the thumb (*1*). The avulsed bone fragment is thus isolated in a medial para-articular position (*2*). Let us recall that the risk of such a manoeuvre during X-raying is the tendinoligamentous interposition or Stener's effect, and the displacement of an unrecognized fracture
3. *Periarthritis* with hydroxyapatite calcification (case 138). This is the same condition we know well in other joints, in particular on the shoulder
4. *Para-articular chondroma.* This is a very uncommon condition. It affects the insertion areas of the articular capsule and the tendon sheaths. The calcifications or ossifications are usually multiple.
5. *Calcified epidermoid cyst.* This is rarely seen, however, in the para-articular area (case 131).

Since the three first possibilities are the most logical, the approach should be:

- Precise history of trauma: bone avulsion
- Pain, even intermittent: periarthritis
- Chance finding during filming: sequel of growth osteochondrosis

143

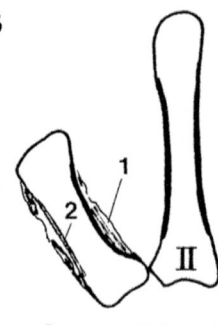

Referred to for trivial trauma, this patient has no history. The radiological anomalies on the first metacarpal are obviously not related to the trauma.

– Periosteal reaction on the entire length of the diaphysis (*1*)
– Minor irregularities in the cortical bone on the radial aspect (*2*)
– The bone piece is otherwise unremarkable

It is thus a *long-standing stabilized lesion* and not a tumour. Two diagnostic possibilities are discussed:

– Osteomyelitis: a discreet form may leave only a simple periosteal reaction; a more advanced form would be accompanied by modifications in the bone itself (sequestration, etc.)
– Tuberculosis: termed spina ventosa, it usually comprises a more voluminous and irregular hyperostostic reaction surrounding the diaphysis.

144

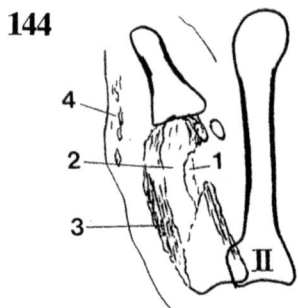

Involvement of the first metacarpal is much more severe:

– Extended osteolysis of the diaphysis and metacarpal head (*1*)
– Sequestration of the central part of the bone (*2*)
– Thick periosteal new bone formation (*3*)
– Unaffected sesamoids
– Thickening of the soft parts with some heterogeneous translucencies about the metacarpophalangeal joint, due to the abscess of the soft parts (*4*)

The diagnosis is, indisputably, *osteomyelitis* of the first metacarpal. This woman had been suffering for 3 weeks from an infection of the thumb which had been incorrectly treated, and had secondarily developed staphylococcic septicaemia.

This finger shows:

– Very marked swelling of the soft parts about the middle and proximal phalanges (*1*)
– Medullary bone rarefaction in the basal part of the middle phalanx (*2*). The subchondral bone is spared and there is no extension to the joint
– The cortex is broken on a large part of the circumference of the bone (*3*) at the same level as the rarefaction

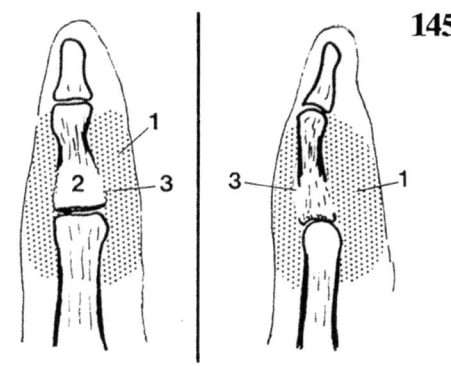

145

We must thus conclude that it is phalangeal *osteitis;* this diagnosis is confirmed by a history of septic prick.

This 17-year-old boy complained about restricted wrist mobility. The clinical examination is normal. The radiograph shows:

– A lucent defect occupying the greater part of the capitate (*1*)
– A sclerotic border surrounding the defect (*2*) with some onset of sequestration
– No rupture of the cortex

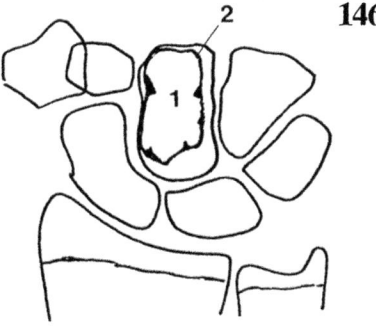

146

Tumours and pseudotumours of the wrist are particularly rare. When there is such a large and tumour-like defect in a carpal bone, one can diagnose a chondroma if the appearance is benign, or a Ewing sarcoma when it is malignant.

However, a large defect, particularly in the capitate or in the hamate, is fairly characteristic of *villonodular synovitis*. This condition often affects young adults and the erosion may involve two adjacent bones, for example, the hamate and the triquetrum. Defects in the cortex can be clearly seen on tomograms.

147

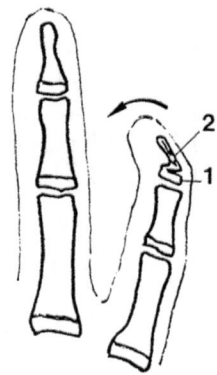

Let us end with a *curiosity*.

This is a *Kirner's deformity*. Of unknown aetiology and rather uncommon, this disease always has the same features: normal epiphysis (*1*) often remaining separate from the diaphysis after the end of growth; and hypoplastic diaphysis with curvature towards the palm (*2*). This anomaly is usually bilateral and involves only the distal phalanx of the fifth finger. It is not accompanied by other disturbances and constitutes only an aesthetic problem. There is of course a relationship with Dupuytren's disease, i.e. retraction of the palmar aponeurosis.

Subject Index